Chasing Pain

T0177534

Chasing Pain

The Search for
a Neurobiological Mechanism

Kenneth L. Casey

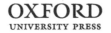

OXFORD
UNIVERSITY PRESS

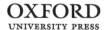

Oxford University Press is a department of the University of Oxford. It furthers
the University's objective of excellence in research, scholarship, and education
by publishing worldwide. Oxford is a registered trade mark of Oxford University
Press in the UK and certain other countries.

Published in the United States of America by Oxford University Press
198 Madison Avenue, New York, NY 10016, United States of America.

© Oxford University Press 2019

CIP data is on file at the Library of Congress
ISBN 978-0-19-088023-1

1 3 5 7 9 8 6 4 2
Printed by Webcom, Inc., Canada

For Jean

CONTENTS

LIST OF ILLUSTRATIONS

FIGURES

TABLES

ACKNOWLEDGMENTS

The Department of Physiology at the University of Washington gave me the opportunity, as a medical student, to experience the excitement of recording the electrophysiological activity of multiple and single neurons from the mammalian somatosensory nervous system. This experience was enhanced under the watchful, thoughtful tutelage of the late Professor Arnold Towe and Dr. Suhayl Jabbur, then a postdoctoral scholar and subsequently a major contributor to the pain research literature. Fred Plum, then the Chief of the Division of Neurology, introduced me to the challenges and opportunities of clinical neurology and provided guided encouragement to complete my clinical training. The late Paul D. MacLean at the National Institutes of Health (Bethesda, Maryland, U.S.A.) introduced me to the limbic system concept and provided me with a unique opportunity to investigate the neurophysiology of pain in the waking mammalian brain. These early experiments were inspired largely by the seminal theories of pain and somatosensory neurophysiology developed by Professors Ronald Melzack and the late Patrick Wall as cited in this book. I am forever indebted to Ron especially for introducing me to the importance of conceptual models as determinants of the direction of research and for guiding our effort to merge the somatosensory and limbic systems into a conceptual model of pain.

I am indebted to Horace Davenport (Chair, Department of Physiology) and Russell DeJong (Chair, Department of Neurology), University of Michigan, for the opportunity to complete my clinical training and to Professors S. Martin Lindenauer and Sid Gilman for the opportunity to continue my career as a physician-neuroscientist as Chief of the Neurology Service at the University-affiliated Veteran's Affairs Medical Center, Ann Arbor, Michigan.

Beyond the support of those cited above, I continue to be encouraged by the scholarly work conducted by my many colleagues in the pain research community and in academic clinical neurology. Their dedication to meeting the challenges presented by painful neurological disorders and by the chase for pain generally is truly inspirational.

Finally, my wife, Jean, stayed with me in the neurophysiology laboratory at the University of Washington during those early years, enduring the usually long, frequently overnight, hours of electrophysiological recording. She later developed an outstanding career in dietetics and has remained a source of inspiration, encouragement, and support throughout our lives together. This book is dedicated to her.

ABOUT THE COVER

The Creation of Pain

The two ovals represent two major processing levels in the central nervous system (spinal cord and brain stem; thalamus and cerebral cortex) and the red arrows represent the interactions among these structures. The lower red arrow represents the somatic and visceral sensory input to the central nervous system (upward direction) and the reflexive and conscious behavioral responses to this input (downward direction). The blue upcurving arrows represent overall environmental influences on pain, including those produced by behavior and cognition.

Access accompanying content at www.oxfordmedicine.com/chasingpain

The copy of *Chasing Pain* you have purchased comes with free access to online video appendices. To access this content, visit www.oxfordmedicine.com/chasingpain.

If you are interested in access to the complete online edition, please consult with your librarian.

INTRODUCTION

WHY PAIN?

No human experience is more important than physical pain, the sensation caused by the physical damage of skin, muscle, bone, or internal organs. Unlike psychological pain, physical pain is experienced as an unpleasant, offensive, often threatening, and sometimes unbearable sensation on or within the body. In its mild to moderate form, pain is a common experience in daily life. But more severe pain is a common and often tenaciously persistent accompaniment of many diseases, including those affecting the organ that creates it, the nervous system.[1] And, unlike many diseases, physical pain usually can be alleviated to some degree—sometimes completely, but often only partially and with undesirable side effects.

Death is preferred over prolonged, severe pain. But even mild to moderate pain, if continued long enough, will bleed life of its pleasure, transforming the individual into a sufferer whose overriding goal is to drive this experience from consciousness. The desire to be rid of or to avoid pain crosses cultural and ethnical boundaries and is at the core of all civil and religious tenets intended to guide behavior through fear of pain. Hell would be much less fearsome without fire.

Tolerating pain is often seen as a virtue. Actions are especially praiseworthy and brave if they lead to the experience or serious threat of pain. The ability to withstand obvious tissue damage without expressing pain is often admired and considered a desirable, even necessary, attribute of manhood, even required as a rite of passage in some tribal societies. Today, billions in international currencies are spent on entertainments, especially sporting events, in which the participants are cheered and rewarded for risking or enduring pain. This reverence for pain derives from the common human experience of its intrinsic unpleasant, sometimes unbearable character.

How can we control it? Throughout the world, a large share of monetary and human resources is devoted to avoiding or eliminating pain. In the United States alone, an estimated 100 million adults suffer persistent, chronic pain, and the annual cost of pain treatment and loss of productivity has been estimated to be within the $500 billion to $600 billion range; this cost estimate does not include television and other advertising expenses for "pain-killing" drugs.[2] Most of the attention to pain has focused on the immediate need for relieving it, especially when it persists beyond the time of healing (chronic pain) or seems unrelated to tissue injury.

Yet, despite our wish to avoid it, we know that pain is essential. Pain usually signals impending or ongoing tissue damage. Physicians rely on a patient's complaint of pain to locate the site of disease or injury and to determine the success or failure of treatments. The rare individuals who lack normal pain sensation suffer unrecognized and untreated injuries, sometimes with fatal consequences.

1

For all of these reasons, pain has been the subject of intense deliberation, discussion, and investigation for centuries. There has also always been, and there remains, a vigorous scientific and philosophical interest in how the experience of pain arises. What are the physical mechanisms that are directly responsible for pain? What is the biology or, more specifically, the *neuro*biology of pain? And what can the neuronal mechanisms of pain tell us about brain function generally? Pain is an experience that arises somewhere in the brain. How does this happen?

Pain is a neurobiological phenomenon. This is a story about researching the neurobiology of pain and the broad implications of that search. The story unfolds chronologically because that is the way science progresses. I have written it with the curious layperson, physician, nurse, or student in mind. I have assumed that the reader has acquired elsewhere a basic knowledge of biology, including some acquaintance with nervous systems. Nonetheless, in proceeding with this story, the reader may wish to review a few neuroscience fundamentals to facilitate understanding the story. If you are not comfortable with your understanding of the basics of neurophysiology and interneuronal communication, you may wish to consider reviewing some of the material in the Appendix before proceeding further. Otherwise, the Appendix can be consulted periodically as needed. Figures in the APPENDIX are referenced in the text as the figure number followed by "A."

THE CHASE

chase (vb): **1a:** *to follow rapidly and intently in order to or as if to trail or overtake, seize, molest, or do violence to:* PURSUE **b:** HUNT **c:** *to follow or attend upon persistently and hopefully with the intention of attracting, alluring, or persuading into companionship or intimacy....*
From *Webster's Third New International Dictionary*.
G. & C. Merriam Company, Springfield, MA, 1971.

This story is about a chase and the broad implications of that chase. The elusive object of the chase is pain: an experience, not an object. Unlike the objects of the chase suggested by the previous definitions, pain cannot be literally overtaken, seized, or molested; and it seems unlikely that one would wish to attract or allure it into intimate companionship. Rather, we chase pain because we wish to control it. And we wish to control it *selectively*, without compromising or interfering with other experiences or body functions.

But an experience cannot be seen, touched, or manipulated. To control something, we usually must understand it in a mechanistic way so that we can manipulate its component parts and determine the direction and intensity of its action or activity. We must give pain some kind of physical substance, at least as a concept in our imagination. That is why this story focuses on the development of a *conceptual model* of pain. Conceptual models are mental representations of how something works. They give abstract concepts like pain something of a physical reality that we can manipulate in our mind so that we might understand how it would function in different conditions, possibly produced by manipulations we might apply. Many of us may not be aware of having a conceptual model, but it is very likely that we have one, whether implicit or explicit, as we approach a task that involves manipulating, investigating, or creating something. We have some expectation of an outcome that is based on our conceptual model. Therefore, conceptual models have serious practical consequences. They determine what we do and how we approach a problem.[3] In the case of pain, a conceptual model determines how a physician or nurse will (or will not) attempt to relieve it, how a researcher will design an experiment to study it, and even how a philosopher will incorporate it into a larger theory of conscious experience.

The first step is to learn as much as we can about it—to lay the foundation for a conceptual model—and that means doing research. Pain research is focused on the acquisition, analysis, and interpretation of data obtained from investigations of human and animal nervous systems, using biochemistry, physiology, anatomy, clinical observations, and an analysis of human and animal behavior. The implicit assumption is that this research will provide a mechanistic understanding of pain. In fact, the research *is* the chase because, once we acquire the critical information about the mechanics of pain, we are at the point of being able to control it, and the chase is essentially over. That's the assumption, anyway.

So, what is the "critical information"? What are we looking for? How will we know when the chase is over? We know that pain emerges from the activity of the nervous system—the brain and the nerves connected to it. We can therefore assume reasonably that pain will emerge from the conjoint activity of connected structures, the nerves in the body that connect to groups of nerve cells that form physically identifiable structures in the brain. This means that we are likely to be looking for nervous system structures that are critical for pain. Any single structure may be necessary but not sufficient for pain and could also be necessary for one or more nonpain functions; however, its membership in the "pain group" would be necessary for pain. To put it simply, *we wish to identify the structures that as a group are necessary and sufficient for pain.* When we find that group, the chase is nearly over, at least to a first approximation. We will still need to investigate the details about how the members of this group interact at the cellular and molecular levels, but an understanding of pain at this systems level will be a major advance and will greatly constrain our conceptual models of pain mechanisms.

The chase for pain began very early in human history, but I will begin following it as it developed during the late 19th century and continues to the present day. Before beginning the story, it is helpful to present some examples of the spectrum of pain-related experiences because this gives us some idea of the territory we must cover to achieve a full and complete mechanistic understanding of pain.

1

A SAMPLE AT THE EXTREMES

PAIN WITHOUT TISSUE DAMAGE

Causalgia

On April 26, 1945, Lee was on patrol with his platoon during the battle of Okinawa. Suddenly, the platoon came under machine gun fire, and a bullet passed through Lee's right thigh, injuring, but not completely severing, his sciatic nerve and partially paralyzing his right leg. He felt the impact of the missile but did not feel pain until two days later, after he had been moved to a field hospital and then to a hospital ship. He was eventually transferred to Oakland Naval Hospital in California, where he came under the care of William K. Livingston, MD, a neurosurgeon whose description of Lee's condition is paraphrased here.[1] The site of Lee's wound was not painful, but he had constant, severe, unbearable burning pain (causalgia) in his *uninjured* right foot. He would not allow anyone to touch the foot and insisted on keeping it in a pail of cool water. The pain was greatly increased by taking a deep breath, by noise created by others around him, by the sound of doors shutting, by music, and even by watching movies. He would not allow his hair to be cut because this increased his pain. He avoided touching dry objects and tried to wet his hands before touching anything. He spent most of each day alone in his bed or in a chair, his foot immersed in water, avoiding contact with other patients or medical staff. He was finally persuaded to begin a rehabilitation program, beginning with foot movements in a water bath. After a year of repeated injections of local anesthetic in the area of the injured nerve and a program of gradual, progressive exercise of his foot, Lee was able to return to duty with only minor sensory loss in his right heel.

Migraine

Terry, a 25-year-old woman, began having headaches at age 12. After several headache spells, which occurred about every two months, she became aware that she could tell when she was about to have a headache. She became sensitive to light, asking for drapes or shades to be closed and wearing sunglasses even on cloudy days. At the same time, she noted that minor noises, like cars going by or planes overhead, would become unpleasant and seem louder than usual. Sometimes, she avoided putting on some types of clothes such as jeans because the texture felt uncomfortably rough and unpleasant. About half an hour after these symptoms, she would note difficulty reading because the central part of her vision was blurred or even missing; the area of visual loss was always surrounded by a band of wavy, colored lights. Within another half hour, she would have severe, throbbing pain behind either her right or left eye. The pain would spread to involve her cheek, forehead, and temple on one side and was sometimes accompanied by nausea and a sense of great fatigue. The headache typically lasted 4 to 6 hours and was not relieved by aspirin or codeine. Physical and neurological examinations were normal. She consulted an otorhinolaryngologist, who irrigated her maxillary sinus, but this had no effect on her headache or other symptoms. Sumatriptan, a medication developed specifically for the migraine syndrome, effectively aborted the headaches if taken orally at the first sign of preheadache symptoms. A bedtime dose of amitriptyline, an antidepressant medication, reduced the frequency of most of these episodes to once or twice a year.

Central Pain

Central pain is given this name because it is generated in the central nervous system and experienced in an uninjured part of the body. In that way, it resembles causalgia, except that there is no injury to a nerve that could be a source of nerve impulses.

Salvatore, a 67-year-old retired investor, suddenly felt a strong "pins and needles" sensation throughout his left body while walking outside; he thinks this did not involve his face. He had a sensation of being unsteady, but no pain or weakness. The next day, he thought that hot and cold water felt less intense on his left side while in the shower; this difference gradually became less noticeable over the next three to four months. A year after his initial symptoms, he developed a dull, aching pain in his left arm and leg and noticed that even mild pressure on that side was painful; even rolling over on that side would awaken him at night. He described the sensation as very unpleasant and "not like normal pain." The constant pain became much worse if he became emotionally upset or was in noisy or brightly lit surroundings. He expressed great concern about the cause of this pain, especially because it appeared long after his initial symptoms. On examination, he had a slightly *elevated* heat detection and heat pain threshold on the left arm and leg but a markedly *reduced* threshold for pressure pain in the same area. Magnetic resonance imaging of the brain revealed a small stroke in the right thalamus (above the spinal cord and below the cerebral cortex). His symptoms were reduced, but not eliminated, by a daily dose of an anticonvulsant medication and a reassuring explanation about the cause of his pain. I told him that the pain was being created in his brain because his stroke had changed the sensory part of his brain; he didn't have a new disease or another stroke, I said. I didn't tell him exactly how all this happened. He wasn't prepared for all that information, and I didn't have the answer, anyway.

A more dramatic example of central pain is that which is sometimes experienced following spinal cord injury. Frequent or nearly constant pain can appear in the legs or sacral area even if the spinal cord is completely severed by trauma or by surgical attempts to stop the pain. An example is presented next, excerpted and slightly shortened from an article that reviewed this condition and estimated that 5% to 10% of patients with this injury experienced this form of central pain.[2]

J.J., a 59-year-old man, had a 33-year history of slowly progressive leg weakness. Severe spasms in the legs were relieved by injecting phenol into the space around the diseased spinal cord. Following this, he complained of burning and aching pain in the right leg and the lower right abdomen. A year later, nerve roots were cut on the right side in an attempt to relieve the pain. This improved the abdominal pain, but there was still pain in the right knee. The following year, a left spinothalamic tract section of the spinal cord was performed in an attempt to relieve the pain. However, eight months later, the patient still reported a great deal of burning pain in the right groin and in the knee. Therefore, a segment of the injured spinal cord was removed (cordectomy). Three years later, the patient again complained of pain around his lower right abdominal area. This had been present for approximately 1 year and was getting worse. At this time it was noted that he had a complete loss of sensation on the right side of his body up to the right nipple, showing that he was complaining of pain in an area of complete sensory loss. Because of the severe pain, another segment of cord was removed completely. After this second cordectomy, it was noted that the patient had increasingly severe pain radiating from his lower right chest into his groin and testicle. It was noted that he had a complete loss of sensation bilaterally below a level just above the nipples. After the cordectomies, bilateral high thoracic local anesthetic blocks were placed at the sympathetic nerve chains adjacent to the spine. There was only a slight improvement in the abdominal and testicular pain and no change at all in the pain in the abdomen and right leg. He died 5 years after the second cordectomy.

TISSUE DAMAGE WITHOUT PAIN

Sports and Ritual Analgesia

Ken, age 19, was on a team playing rugby against a rugged group from Vancouver, BC. Shortly after a particularly vigorous scrum, in which the two teams tightly bunch up together and fight for the ball placed between them, the ball went out of bounds, and the referee stopped play. The teams then lined up perpendicular to the sideline (a "line out"), and the referee prepared to throw the ball inbounds; he then stopped, pointed at Ken, and announced: "Your ear's about off!" Ken's right side was covered with blood dripping from an ear that was partially ripped from the side of his head. He felt no pain until the nurse at the infirmary cleaned it with alcohol and bound the ear to his head with a bandage. The wound healed naturally without complications.

This personal account is a very minor example of common sports analgesia.[3] I'm confident, however, that under almost any other circumstance, I would have yelled out in pain and grabbed the side of my head. However, during every football, ice hockey, or other sports season, one can observe numerous examples of this phenomenon as players get up and continue playing soon after collisions and other injuries that would have immobilized them for a much longer time if sustained outside the arena of competition.

What I am calling "sports analgesia" is similar to *ritual analgesia*, during which normally painful injuries are sustained while the subject is in what could be called a state of rapture. For example, in the Mandan Native American culture in what is now North Dakota, groups of young men were expected to participate in the secret Okipa Earth-creation ceremony in which, after fasting for several days, and surrounded by much chanting, dancing, and drumming, they allowed wooden skewers to be pierced through the skin of their back, arms, and legs and were hung by the skin of their backs from the top of the ceremonial lodge. While suspended for many hours, buffalo skulls were hung from the skewers in their legs. Expressions of pain were considered shameful. If the men lost consciousness during this torture, as most did, they were brought down and allowed to recover, a sign of spiritual acceptance. Between Okipa ceremonies, and usually before hunts or battles, male Mandans often fasted for days, hung themselves from trees or embankments, or severed fingers in hopes of experiencing a vision or receiving a favorable spiritual signal.[4] In its contemporary, gentler form, hanging by one's skin is an elaborate, organized affair, practiced by groups of devotees of body modification, tattooing, and skin piercing.[5] Suspension of the body by skin hooks is an ancient practice, but in the early Mandan, as well as current practices, it appears that the participant achieves and, more critically, *expects* to achieve, a state of euphoria that profoundly attenuates or eliminates the pain normally expected under these circumstances (see URL link in Figure 1.1). A high degree of self-selection and group encouragement seems to be important also. Perhaps this isn't as painful as it looks (see Figure 1.1), but don't try this at home.

Surgery Without Anesthesia

Today, both local and general anesthetics are administered before and during surgery—and for good reason. Before the discovery and development of general, regional, and local anesthesia in the mid-19th century, surgery was a horrible procedure, dreaded by both patient and surgeon. Martin Pernick gives numerous graphic accounts of the agony of preanesthesia surgery and how surgeons of the day were trained to ignore the screams of their patients.[6] Yet long before this era, there were examples of surgery being performed while the patient showed no signs of pain. In his book on cross-cultural comparisons of attitudes about pain, Eric Hayot cites numerous examples of both torture and surgery in the absence of expressions of pain.[7] In this book, Hayot refers to the phenomenon of "acupuncture anesthesia" as witnessed by, among others, the Acupuncture Anesthesia Study Group (AASG) in a visit to China in May 1974. To better understand the phenomenon of anesthetic-free surgery and why it should influence our understanding of the neurophysiology of pain, I will detour here to offer a brief account of my personal experiences as a member of the AASG.

Notes from China, 1974: The Acupuncture Anesthesia Study Group

On International Worker's Day (May 1, 1974), our train from Hong Kong left the transfer point at Lo Wu and entered the People's Republic of China (PRC); the Cultural Revolution was still in place. Our delegation, the AASG,[8] was to determine the effectiveness of acupuncture in preventing or relieving the pain of surgery. We were among several other "people-to-people" exchanges that took place since Henry Kissinger and President Richard Nixon visited the PRC and met with Chairman Mao Tse-tung (1971–1972) before the establishment of formal diplomatic relationships between the United States and the PRC. Our report has been published by the National Academy of Sciences (1976),[9] and the full text is available here (https://books.google.com/books?id=UjQrAAAAYA AJ&lpg=PR1&dq=inauthor%3A%22American%20Acupuncture%20Anesthesia%20 Study%20Group%22&pg=PP1#v=onepage&q&f=false).

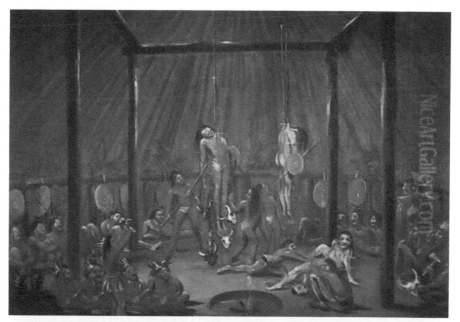

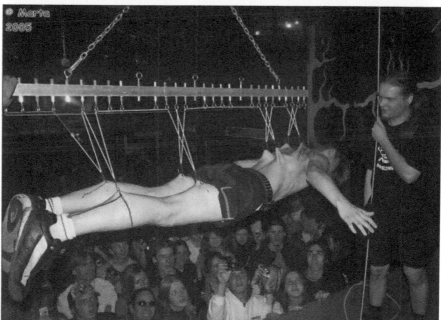

FIGURE 1.1. Ritual analgesia. *Top*: The Mandan Okipa ceremony. See text for description. (https://commons.wikimedia.org/wiki/File:%27The_Cutting_Scene,_Mandan-O-kee-pa_Ceremony%27,_oil_on_canvas_painting_by_George_Catlin,_1832.jpg). *Bottom*: Body suspension demonstration. Interviews with participants indicate that they feel pain when the hooks are inserted but that the pain is reduced or absent as they experience a state of euphoria during the suspension.

Our AASG observed surgical procedures performed without the use of general or regional anesthesia. Acupuncture anesthesia is a misleading phrase because there is not a global loss of sensation or of consciousness; rather, there is a loss, or at least a significant and selective attenuation, of pain during surgery with acupuncture. *Acupuncture hypalgesia* (AH; reduced pain) would be a more accurate description of the condition we were sent to observe. Although acupuncture and other forms of counter-irritation have been used for centuries,[10] it has only been since the late 1950s that major surgeries were performed using acupuncture as the primary or even exclusive method of preventing surgical pain. Encouraging the use of AH in surgery became part of the postrevolutionary national effort, guided by Chairman Mao, to demonstrate the superiority, or at least equivalence, of traditional Chinese medicine (TCM) over Western medical practice. AH is, or was, a modern, postrevolutionary derivative of TCM, practiced largely to enhance China's image as an important contributor to modern medical science and practice.[11,12]

Over the next three weeks, our group visited 16 hospitals in four cities (Beijing, Shanghai, Guangzhou, and Hangzhou) and witnessed 48 surgeries performed with AH for pain control. We were nearly always granted permission, by the patients and surgeons, to film the operation.

Before beginning our observations in the PRC, we developed a checklist to document our observations and a system for grading the effectiveness of AH. We were aware of the problem of using behavioral observations and physiological measurements (changes in heart rate, blood pressure, and respiration) to judge the hypalgesic effect of acupuncture. We realized that the patients we were about to observe could experience varying degrees of pain that, for whatever reason, would escape the detection of the anesthesiologists, neurological clinicians, and neuroscientists in our group. Nonetheless, because the realities of daily life and medical practice compel us to make judgments about pain, we employed a grading system similar to that used by our Chinese colleagues, summarized as follows:

Grade 1: No behavioral or physiological signs of pain and no use of local anesthetics
Grade 2: Mild or transient indications of pain with or without the injection of local anesthetic in doses insufficient to account for the analgesic effect
Grade 3: Frequent signs of pain with or without the use of local anesthesia
Grade 4: Signs of pain throughout the procedure and frequent use of local anesthesia

On May 4, 1974, at what was then called the Third Beijing General Hospital, I filmed the removal of a noncancerous thyroid tumor (thyroid adenoma) from a healthy-appearing 30-year-old woman. She had received a preoperative intramuscular sedative dose (50 milligrams) of meperidine, an opioid analgesic used for mild to moderate pain, about an hour before surgery. No other anesthetic or analgesic medications were used before or during this surgery. As shown in Figure 1.2,[13] she appears alert and fully responsive throughout the surgery.

For approximately 10 to 20 minutes before the incision, electrical stimulation was applied through acupuncture needles placed in the neck and ear; this appeared to be painless. Throughout the surgery, the patient's face, seen behind the operative field barrier,

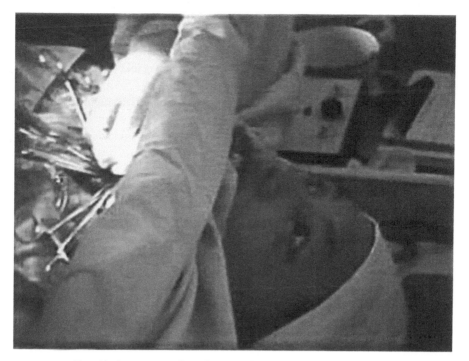

FIGURE 1.2. Thyroid adenectomy performed using only acupuncture as an analgesic agent at the Third Beijing General Hospital, May 4, 1974.

showed no behavioral evidence of pain. The anesthesiologist in our group detected no changes in blood pressure or respiration. Given the extent of tissue damage and manipulation, as well as common clinical experience, the degree of apparent analgesia shown here is not explained by the preoperative dose of meperidine, although this may have facilitated natural physiological mechanisms of analgesia.

An ovarian cyst was removed from a 30-year-old woman who had experienced two months of menstrual irregularity and intermittent abdominal pain. I obtained this and related clinical information from Dr. Chang, the gynecological surgeon, who spoke nearly flawless English. The late Ephriam ("Rick") Siker, MD, chairman of the Department of Anesthesiology, Mercy Hospital, University of Pittsburgh, was with me throughout this surgery and was allowed to assist in monitoring the patient's blood pressure and respiratory reactions during the operation. I have inserted here, in italics, excerpts from my dictation on the day of surgery (May 4, 1974; Third Beijing General Hospital).

The patient was told that she would have acupuncture for analgesia because (it) is routinely offered to patients for removal of ovarian cysts. I asked Dr. Chang what would happen if the patient refused (acupuncture analgesia), and I was told that she would be offered conventional anesthesia or preferably spinal block. The patient was apparently not prepared for (acupuncture analgesia) in any other way except that she was told about the details of the operation . . . and what would happen in the operating room. According to Dr. Chang, there was no encouragement for participating in acupuncture analgesia, and the patient apparently did not know, nor did Dr. Chang, that we were going to be here to observe this procedure.

I did not determine whether this patient had been given preoperative testing with acupuncture needling as is often done. As in the thyroid adenectomy shown earlier, the patient received 50 milligrams of meperidine by intramuscular injection about an hour before entering the operating room. Acupuncture stimulation needles were placed in her back, abdomen, and legs, all without local or general anesthetics. Electrical stimulation was applied through these needles for about 20 minutes before the surgery began. Local anesthetics were not used at any time. During the surgery, there was no facial or other behavioral evidence for pain. Dr. Siker was unable to detect any pain-related changes in blood pressure or respiration during this surgery. Immediately after the surgery, I took the opportunity to perform a brief examination with the help of one of the Chinese translators who accompanied us. The patient was able to move all limbs normally and distinguish light touch from pinprick in the legs and lower abdomen, consistent with the absence of spinal or regional anesthetic block.

On May 6, at the Beijing Tuberculosis Research Institute, a 41-year-old man had a partial pulmonary lobectomy performed for an old tuberculous cavity in the right upper lobe. He had previously experienced some coughing of blood and had a positive sputum culture for the tubercle bacillus. This patient received no preoperative analgesic medicine. Acupuncture needles were placed on the chest and in the right hand, which was supported above his face while an acupuncturist manipulated the needle continuously throughout the surgery.

After electrical stimulation through the acupuncture needles (about 15 to 20 minutes), the incision was made, followed by dissection through the chest muscles. The patient did not move or change his facial expression at any time. Our anesthesiologist (Dr. Jerome Modell, University of Florida, Gainesville) noted:

> [A]t the time the incision was made, his (pulse and blood pressure) did not change after the incision was made and within approximately 2 or 3 minutes after the incision. We paid particular attention to the vital signs and his facial expressions at the time they made the incision when he did not react, when they applied voltage, and at this time he did say that he felt some heat from the coagulating current. We paid attention at the time they placed the rib spreader and there was really no change in his vital signs until the hemothorax (blood in the chest cavity) was created. At that point, his respiratory rate went from 18 to possible [*sic*] 24 . . . but his vital signs (remained) in a very respectable area.

During the surgery (about 70 minutes), the patient used his abdominal and diaphragmatic muscles to expand his left lung. He received supplementary oxygen for several minutes through a mask suspended about an inch over his face after his chest was opened. I did not photograph the entire operation, but the video (see note 16) shows part of the wound closure toward the end of surgery. Dr. Modell summarized: "This was a 100% success."

Summarizing the Conclusions of the Acupuncture Anesthesia Study Group

The surgeries we observed ranged from tooth extractions to major thoracic and abdominal operations. Details are available in the original report. In summary, most of our group (see the exception given later) agreed that grades 1 and 2 represented the degree of pain control that would be acceptable in the United States, and we placed 35 (73%) of the 48 surgeries in these categories. The remaining 13 surgeries (27%) were considered unacceptable and given grades 3 or 4. In our report, we noted that "even in China, AH has relatively limited application since only some 15% of all patients are selected for this type of pain control" (p. 28). Based on our sample observations, we estimated that only 10% of the total surgical population could be expected to experience adequate pain control. In our concluding comments (p. 30), we noted further that "AH is a significant human biological phenomenon of unknown mechanisms. The induction of a hypnotic trance is not necessary. Social factors may be important in some instances but are not, of themselves, sufficient to account for the effects observed. *Some psychophysiological process appears to be important in modifying the experience of pain*" (italics mine). We emphasized that AH was in the experimental stage and that further studies were necessary before it could be considered for use in Western medicine (p. 28).

In a note to our conclusions, our report acknowledged that Arthur Taub, MD, PhD, dissented from these conclusions and referenced an article he authored in *Yale Medicine,* vol. 9, pp. 4–6, 1974 (not available here). I have copied in the following excerpt a transcript of a taped sample of his remarks to the group at our concluding meeting on May 21, 1974. This excerpt is intended to reflect his overall judgment about AH as he observed it during our visit.

> I have seen patients deny pain after the surgery but . . . I do not believe them. I believe that all human beings are alike and when they are subjected to surgical trauma they suffer pain. Now, whether they express it or not in a dictatorship is a matter for people to discuss. . . . I submit to you that the majority of patients who manifested minimal suffering in fact received, even though it appeared gross, minimal trauma to nociceptors and that those people who did suffer received greater trauma to nociceptors. They have been coerced. They have been coerced to perform (these) operations.[14]

Dr. Taub's comment represents the view that pain depends entirely on the amount of tissue damage and the excitation of tissue receptors that are uniquely sensitive to this damage (nociceptors). According to this interpretation, the patients undergoing surgeries we graded as 1 or 2, including those shown in the videos here, experienced pain during surgery but withheld behavioral and even physiological evidence for it because of political or cultural coercion. In a recent article,[15] Dr. Taub maintained this view of AH but agreed that "some major surgical procedures have been performed in China using only small amounts of premedication, little or no local anesthetic, and the insertion of acupuncture needles. Surgical procedures that have been witnessed have gone well, but postoperative studies have not been done."

The Acupuncture Anesthesia Study Group: A Retrospective

In his Appendix of original translations from the Chinese,[16] Paul Unschuld reprinted an article by clinicians Keng Hsi-chen and T'ao Nai-huang that appeared approximately 5 years after the Cultural Revolution on October 22, 1980, in the Chinese newspaper *Wen-hui pao* under the title, *The Examination of Acupuncture Anesthesia Must Seek Truth from Facts*. In this article, the authors state that they have "in the past, from 1969 through 1977 . . . conducted more than thirty thousand surgical operations under acupuncture anesthesia as an exploratory practice in order to wholeheartedly promote acupuncture anesthesia." They observe that "the suppression of pain is incomplete" during AH and that "excellent results (are achieved in) at the most merely 60 to 85 percent [of the cases], while in 15 to 40% the results are not good or are even a failure." They note that "[d]uring the period of the Cultural Revolution . . . physicians and patients were under the pressure of the political requirements of that time." Although they state that "in some sections of surgery, acupuncture anesthesia is still effective, such as in surgery on thyroid glands," they emphasize the limited applications of AH and encourage more systematic studies of its use in the absence of political or cultural influences.

The article by Keng and T'ao largely confirms the observations of the AASG but also gives partial support to Taub's assertion that some patients were withholding expressions of pain because of political and cultural constraints. There is no doubt that the application of AH was a consequence of the political climate during the Cultural Revolution.[17] It is notable that the application of AH has declined substantially since the Cultural Revolution, although it is difficult to obtain information about this point. Recent reviews and reports indicate that the use of AH is infrequent and limited to a select group of relatively brief and uncomplicated surgeries.[18]

Nonetheless, it may be difficult for most observers to accept the argument that the surgeries inflicted trauma so minimal as to avoid completely the pain of tissue damage most of us experience in daily life, especially after seeing the videos (see end note 13). To test this possibility, some members of the AASG purchased an electroacupuncture stimulator and, using a stimulation protocol we had observed recently, attempted to produce AH in one of our colleagues in one of our hotel rooms in the PRC. Our intrepid volunteer was unable to tolerate even pinpricks within the "operative field." It would also be difficult to convince most observers that the surgical patients we categorized in groups 1 and 2 were simply cooperating with Chairman Mao by voluntary, even heroic, behavioral restraint. There seems to be more to AH than simple political or cultural coercion.

SUMMARIZING THIS SAMPLE
OF PAIN-RELATED EXPERIENCES

The samples presented in this chapter are intentionally unrepresentative of the pain or analgesia experienced by healthy individuals in the course of daily living. The mechanisms that mediate more ordinary pain-related experiences will be discussed later along with some other rare, genetically based examples of disconnections between pain and tissue damage. For now, I am simply suggesting a range of normal human experiences that a complete conceptual model of pain mechanisms should cover.

There is a common feature among the examples of pain without tissue damage. In each case, the individual experiences an increase in pain when exposed to some normally nonpainful stimuli such as a touches, sounds, or lights. In some examples, these events actually trigger the onset of pain; in others, the ongoing pain is increased by emotional upsets, even minor ones. In the cases of causalgia and central pain, damage to the nervous system has created pain in an uninjured part of the body, a condition now called "neuropathic pain", which will be discussed in subsequent chapters. In the patient with migraine headache, however, there is no evidence of damage to either neural or extraneural tissues. Nonetheless, at least under the pathological conditions represented by these cases, neural mechanisms mediating that normally determine the presence and intensity of pain have been changed so that so that normally painless sensory, emotional, and cognitive functions generate and amplify pain.

By contrast, those with painless or nearly painless tissue damage appear to be, at least in these examples, in a physiological condition that depends not on disease or injury but rather on a cognitive state with a strong focus on attaining a highly desirable goal or reward. In the case of sports analgesia, the focus is obviously on victory over the opponent and possibly the accolades (and various desirable forms of personal attention) anticipated by that victory. In ritual analgesia, the anticipated reward may be the reception of spiritual blessings or, in its modern form, the attainment of a state of bliss unrealizable in ordinary life. The cognitive state associated with analgesia or hypalgesia during surgery with acupuncture alone is more difficult, perhaps impossible, to characterize satisfactorily. However, from the evidence available then and in the years following the Cultural Revolution in the PRC, it seems safe to suggest that unusually strong, historically enriched, cultural influences led many patients and surgeons to have the confident expectation that acupuncture, an important component of TCM, would provide a degree of pain control necessary to eliminate or greatly reduce the pain of surgery. In that sense, surgical AH, sports analgesia, and ritual analgesia have in common an expectation, conscious or otherwise, that pain will be very much in the background. Here again, as in the cases of pain without tissue damage, neural processes that underlie cognitive states have access to mechanisms that modify pain.

2

DRIVERS OF PAIN RESEARCH AND
A MEETING IN ISSAQUAH

There are many reasons for conducting pain research, but I have selected three main categories that seem to include most of the main implicit and explicit goals of this endeavor. Clearly, these drivers of pain research overlap considerably and are certainly not exclusive of one another.

MEDICINE

The psychological, medical, and economic significance of pain is reason enough to invest substantial human and capital resources in research on its causes and treatment. If all pain, especially persistent, chronic pain, could be prevented or treated adequately, the savings, in both human and monetary terms, would be considerable. Aside from prevention, the holy grail of pain treatment is the development of an ideal analgesic. The ideal analgesic would provide complete pain relief without addiction or other unwanted side effects, have a controlled site and duration of action, and would be safe, inexpensive, and easy to administer. We remain far from this goal, but the possibility of reaching it keeps the chase alive.

NEUROSCIENCE

Neuroscience is the study of nervous systems: how they are constructed and organized to explore the world and to survive in hostile environments. At one level, neuroscience is an intellectual exercise similar to investigating how a clock works. The physical, chemical, and cellular machinery of a nervous system may be studied without consideration for anything beyond understanding a limited endpoint function such as the detection of a chemical or light or the execution of a movement. At another level, neuroscience has an explicit goal, such as improving some specific function like mobility or determining the cause of a disease that affects nervous systems. And at still another level, the goal of all neuroscience is to understand how brains, and specifically human brains, perform all the functions that can be identified—from relatively simple reflexive behaviors to complex cognitive tasks. There are many potentially fruitful avenues of approach to all these levels of investigation, but the study of pain, particularly the neural mechanisms responsible for it, happens to lead naturally to each and all of them. Pain is unique among sensory experiences because it has a dominant and defining affective or hedonic[1] component that is unpleasant and triggers efforts to relieve, escape, and avoid it. Even the brief, mild pain from a needle, a thorn, or a rock in your shoe has this negative hedonic quality; and pain that is more severe and prolonged often has serious behavioral consequences, such as misdirected anger, depression, and even suicide. Without this affective component, pain would not be pain; it would simply be another sensation that would incidentally inform you about tissue damage that you could choose to ignore. Instead, the "hurt" of pain drives us to action and triggers memory functions that enable us to avoid it in the future. Because pain has this intrinsic affective quality, understanding the neurophysiology of pain could give us a more complete understanding of the neural mechanisms that underlie feeling states generally.

PHILOSOPHY

Pain emerges only from the conscious brain. A deep understanding of the neurophysiology of pain could bring an equally deep and broad understanding of brain function generally, including the neurophysiology of consciousness. The neuroscientific and philosophical literature on consciousness typically includes references to pain as an example of a high level of self-awareness because it is experienced on or within the body. If we could specify the exact anatomical and chemical brain condition that causes pain, we would also be specifying the neurophysiology of a particular subset of conscious experiences, potentially leading to a mechanistic understanding of consciousness itself. The possibility of ever achieving this deep mechanistic understanding has long been, and continues to be, a subject of intense debate. We are certainly farther from this goal than from the medical one, but the possibility of success remains a driving incentive. Collectively, humans have an intense desire to understand themselves and their universe. Like understanding the cosmos, understanding the neural mechanisms of consciousness may have few immediate societal benefits, but the long-term effects may be even more profound than the medical ones. Our world might be a more hospitable and sustainable place if we all embraced the concept of a common neurobiological foundation for each human's personal experience and behavior.

A MEETING IN ISSAQUAH

In late May 1973, about 340 researchers and clinicians from 14 countries sequestered themselves for 6 days in a semi-wilderness area near Issaquah, Washington, a small town 20 miles east of Seattle. They met in what was then called the Providence Convention Center, a largely depopulated campus of the Sisters of Providence, a Catholic nursing order. Meeting attendees were quartered in the rather austere accommodations of the vacant campus dormitories; there was no publically available transportation outside the Center. In the near distance, one could see nuns walking among the few other buildings on the campus.

We had been summoned to this remote location by John J. Bonica, MD (1917–1994), then Professor and Chair of Anesthesiology at the University of Washington and author of a seminal book, *The Management of Pain* (Lea & Febiger, 1953). John Bonica was a personally and professionally persuasive physician with an international reputation based largely on his development of regional anesthetic methods such as epidural and spinal anesthesia. Many of his techniques and approaches to pain management were developed during World War II, when he was stationed at Fort Lewis, near Tacoma, Washington. John's familiarity with pain was both personal and professional. He was a unique combination of physically impressive athlete (championship amateur and professional wrestling), uncompromising scholar-clinician, and charming, charismatic leader. The fact that he was known to have been born on an island just off the Sicilian coast and spoke with a slight Brooklyn-Italian accent gave him an especially commanding presence. When John summoned, one listened.

At the time of the Issaquah meeting (aka: International Symposium on Pain), research on or about pain lacked a cohesive forum for the presentation of research and discussion of issues related to medical practice or neuroscience. Pain research was conducted and published only as part of a historically established discipline such as anesthesiology, neurophysiology, psychology, or other subdisciplines of biology and health care. John Bonica, however, considered chronic pain a disease, deserving its own special place in the medical literature with an allocation of the appropriate financial and human resources for research. John's call to arms occurred just as new contributions in pain research piqued the intense interest of scientists and clinicians. A new theory about the neurophysiological mechanism of pain had been published eight years earlier, followed shortly by the discovery of nerve fibers that responded only to stimuli that were likely to be painful. These publications provided contrasting and hotly debated views about the mechanisms underlying the perception of pain and raised new questions about pain treatment.

The semi-wilderness meeting near Issaquah reflected John Bonica's goal of establishing an international organization to promote and support pain research and improve pan treatment throughout the world. Buoyed by the excitement of the new salience of pain research, the Issaquah assembly voted to sustain the visibility and impact of pain research and practice by forming the International Association for the Study of Pain (IASP).[2]

At the time of the Issaquah meeting, recent research and emerging concepts were generating debates, sometimes quite heated ones, about the neural mechanisms mediating pain. Does the activity of a single, anatomically or biochemically identifiable group of nerve fibers or nerve cells cause pain *and pain alone*? Or does pain arise from some complex, possibly unrecognizable pattern of activity among the nerve fibers and billions of brain cells that also participate in other functions? These questions are the subjects of debate today and are not simply arcane, academic arguments. The answers to these questions or the ideas about them strongly influence and frequently determine clinical practices aimed at relieving pain. The development of analgesic drugs, the use of medical devices, and the performance of various invasive surgical procedures are all based on an explicit or implicit *conceptual model* of how pain arises from nerve impulses in the body and from the activity of nerve cells in the brain. Conceptual models of pain mechanisms can lead to practical, effective approaches to relieving the many forms of pain encountered in everyday life and in the clinic; but they may also encourage practices that are wasteful of human and monetary resources and are potentially or actually harmful. *Primum non nocere!*[3]

CONCEPTUAL MODELS OF PAIN AT ISSAQUAH (1973)

Why, at the time of the Issaquah meeting, was there a heightened interest in pain and its underlying neural mechanisms? The main reason for the timing of the Issaquah meeting and for the attendance of so many scientists and clinicians is that the study of nervous systems, and especially research on pain, was undergoing unprecedented growth based on the interest generated by research during the preceding decade. The Society for Neuroscience (SfN) had just been formed (1969) and had held its first meeting (1971) with more than 1400 attendees.[4] Highlighting the new salience of pain research, this new society elected Edward Perl (1926–2014) as its first (acting) president. Guided by evidence from pioneering experiments conducted over the previous four decades,[5] Dr. Perl led research showing that some single skin nerve fibers innervate receptors that respond primarily or exclusively to stimuli that would normally be painful when applied to human skin.[6] These skin receptors generate action potentials in the thinnest (small-diameter) nerve fibers, which have little or no axonal myelin and therefore have the slowest action potential conduction velocities and the highest thresholds for electrical stimulation among all other nerve fibers. (By contrast, the large-diameter heavily myelinated nerve fibers innervating tactile [touch] or joint receptors have the lowest electrical stimulation thresholds.) The technical difficulty of recording action potentials from thin, small-diameter fibers prompted theories of pain mechanisms that assumed their absence. Eventually, these receptors came to be known as nociceptors ("noxious receptors"), a term first suggested, mostly on theoretical grounds, by the English neurophysiologist, Sir Charles Sherrington (1857–1952).

Slightly before the discovery of nociceptors, a psychologist, Ronald Melzack (1929–), and a neurophysiologist, Patrick Wall (1925–2001), published a new theory of pain mechanisms[7] based on what was then weaker evidence for the existence of nociceptors and the emerging neurophysiological evidence that mechanisms in the brain and spinal cord (central nervous system, or CNS) controlled or "gated" sensory input to the spinal cord. The "gate control" theory of Melzack and Wall proposed that pain and pain intensity were determined by the activity of a mixture of physiologically distinct large- and small-diameter sensory fibers and by impulses descending from the brain to sensory neurons in the spinal cord; it emphasized the variability of pain and particularly the clinical observations[8] that pain intensity often failed to correlate with the degree of tissue damage.

The terms "nociceptor" and "gate control" could be considered opposing ends of a spectrum of ideas about pain at the Issaquah meeting. The term "nociceptor" attempts to avoid the suggestion that the experience of pain invariably results when nociceptors are stimulated, but the suggestion is probably unavoidable nonetheless. The term "nociceptor" conjures in the casual mind the concept that pain is inextricably linked to a fully deterministic peripheral sensory apparatus. Thus, there are "pain receptors" and "pain fibers." To the clinician, this concept could mean that the nociceptor is the only reasonable target for pain relief. To the researcher, this concept might lead to de-emphasizing or even ignoring other important determinants of perceived pain intensity. The concept of "gate control," by contrast, tends to dissociate pain from the activation of sensory receptors by emphasizing that a complex neurophysiology underlies pain and that the

CNS controls sensation. "Gate control" argues that numerous variables affect pain; but this leads to a level of uncertainty that discomforts clinicians and researchers. Simplicity brings the comfort of clarity and guidance for research and clinical practice, whereas complexity raises bothersome questions at every turn. The bumper-sticker shorthand for these contrasting ideas was, and remains, "specificity versus pattern." At the core of this debate is the question of the degree to which human experience is determined by the peripheral or central nervous systems. In a sense, it is the old "nature versus nurture" argument in a neurological context.

However, at the time of the Issaquah meeting, the background for pain research and treatment consisted of far more than nociceptors and gate control. The specificity-pattern debate was energized by recent findings and theories, but pain had been the subject of observation, research, and philosophical debate for centuries. Several much older concepts also formed the foundation of contemporary medical practice and research.

3

FUNCTIONAL LOCALIZATION, THE SPINOTHALAMIC TRACT, AND NEUROSURGERY FOR PAIN

FUNCTIONAL LOCALIZATION

During the late 18th century and throughout the 19th century, observations of the effects of various neurological lesions in animals and humans suggested that certain specific neurological functions could be physically located within the brain.[1] Thus, it became evident that lesions within some of the components of the central nervous system (CNS) led to clinically identifiable deficits in human behavior. Destruction of parts of the spinal cord and brainstem produced severe sensory and motor impairments while sparing consciousness, language, and cognitive functions. For example, cerebellar damage predominantly affected coordination and gait, occipital lobe lesions produced a variety of specific visual deficits, and damage to the brain's parietal and frontal lobes impaired sensory and motor functions on the opposite side of the body. These early observations led to the concept that identifiable neurological functions were mediated by grossly localizable areas of the CNS.

An extreme example of the functional localization idea was phrenology, a concept proposed by Franz Joseph Gall (1758–1828) in the early 1800s. Gall and his colleague, Johan Spurzheim, believed that human characteristics such as destructiveness, wisdom, acquisitiveness, passion, humor, and many others were produced by localized enlargements within the convoluted cortex of the brain's surface; these cortical enlargements were thought to produce palpable bumps on the skull. A skilled phrenologist was supposed to be able to discern a person's character by careful palpation of the skull.

Gall's extreme localization concept was not widely accepted by the contemporary scientific or religious communities. Therefore, the assignment of neurological functions to specific brain loci remained in the background until 1861 when Pierre Paul Broca (1824–1880) published his clinical observation that damage restricted to the left hemisphere severely affected the production of speech. The critical location of this lesion, in the ventral posterior part of the left frontal lobe, became known as "Broca's area." Carl Wernicke (1848–1905) later (1874) reported that lesions located posterior to Broca's area degraded the comprehension, but not the production of spoken language. Other examples of anatomically localizable functions were described during this period, including partial blindness following damage of the posterior (occipital) cortex and the identification of a "motor" cortex by electrical stimulation and focal lesion studies in animals. Because of these and other related clinical examples, the concept of functional localization became widely recognized as a fundamental organizing principle of the nervous system and has been a major determinant of the direction of neurological research and medical practice. However, a more detailed analysis of additional experiments and subsequent clinical observations raised questions about how fundamental neurological functions are defined, how they are distinguished from symptoms or signs of disease or injury, the degree of anatomical precision with which functions are localized, and how this localization is produced by neurons. These and related unanswered questions remain the focus of intense debate today.

The concept of functional localization profoundly influenced the practice of medicine, especially the treatment of pain. For some of the early philosophers, pain was a disembodied spirit or quale that somehow infused the body but was not part of it. Others assigned pain to the heart or other organs. The concept of the brain as the mediator of pain was not taken seriously until the Greco-Roman physician and philosopher, Galen (130–200), argued, in his treatise, *De usu partium*, that the brain was the source of all ideas and received all sensations. Later, as anatomical dissection and analysis developed, concepts about pain were derived primarily from observations of pain or analgesia as a consequence of disease or injury.[2] Severing nerves to relieve pain probably dates back to the 16th and 17th centuries.[3] However, it soon became obvious that this procedure also caused the loss of other body (somatic) sensations such as touch and temperature, and, when the nerve contained both motor and sensory fibers, there was an added impairment or loss of movement. Practitioners of healing also saw that the destruction of parts of the spinal cord or brain were known to cause an attenuation, a complete loss, or changes in the quality of other sensations, including pain.

THE SPINOTHALAMIC TRACT

Beginning in the mid-19th century, surgical lesion experiments on animals suggested that cutting fibers in the white matter of the spinal cord could reduce or eliminate behavioral responses to noxious (usually painful) stimulation while sparing responses to innocuous tactile stimuli. In experiments on a variety of mammals, the physician-scientist Charles-Edouard Brown-Sequard (1817–1894) showed that a knife slice through one half of the spinal cord (perpendicular to its long axis) reduced behavioral responses to noxious stimulation of the hindlimb on the side of the body below and *opposite* the side of the lesion while sparing responses to noxious stimulation of the hindlimb on the operated side. This result supported Brown-Sequard's hypothesis that a sensory pathway for pain crossed the midline within the spinal cord below the level of the surgical cut before ascending toward the brain. Brown-Sequard also reported on clinical cases of spinal cord damage in which painful and thermal sensations were diminished on the side of the body below and opposite the damaged spinal cord site; tactile and "muscle sense" sensations, however, were spared and seemed to depend on impulses transmitted by separate pathways in the dorsal (posterior) part of the spinal cord. Taken together, these observations were widely accepted as evidence for a distinct, crossed pain- and temperature-sensing pathway to the brain, one that is separate from pathways for touch and other body sensations. This concept of the organization of somatic sensory pathways in the spinal cord is taught in medical schools today.

The results of Brown-Sequard's experiments were not quite so simple, however, as he reported in an 1849 update of his observations[4]:

> Since [the 1846 report], I have had occasion to do this experiment more than 60 times. . . . This is what I have seen:
>
> 1. *Immediately* after cutting a lateral half of the cord in the dorsal region of a mammal, sensation appears very diminished in the hindlimb of the side of the section. Feeling is completely lacking in the other hindlimb. Sometimes, I have found sensation intact or nearly so in the lower limb corresponding to the side of the section, while the opposite hindlimb was either insensitive or very slightly sensitive. [italics mine]
>
> 2. After five to ten minutes of rest following the operation, one always finds the hindlimb corresponding to the side of the section very sensitive. In many cases, or even in most cases, this limb appears noticeably more sensitive than normal. This fact is certainly very curious; but there is another fact, even more unexpected: the hindlimb of the side opposite the section is insensitive or very slightly sensitive.
>
> It follows from these facts that cutting a lateral half of the spinal cord, far from causing loss of sensation in the parts caudad to the section on the same side, renders them hyperesthetic. At the same time, a more or less complete anesthesia is produced on the other side of the body, caudad to the section.

These hemisections of the spinal cord also caused impairment of voluntary movements below and on the side of the lesion; this, however, was not then considered in the analysis of sensory functions.

Thus, Brown-Sequard discovered not only that a crossed sensory pathway mediated responses to noxious stimulation but that responsiveness on the side below the lesion was actually increased. At the time, it could not be determined whether this increased responsiveness was due only to exaggerated reflexive motor responses to the sensory stimulation or included an enhancement of sensory input. Later, however, Brown-Sequard reported his clinical observation that, in humans, the sensations of tickling and temperature were greatly increased below and on the same side as the spinal lesion.[5] It was thus clear that spinal cord lesions could cause increased as well as decreased neuronal excitability. The fact that this excitability increase occurred below, and not above, the cord lesion suggested that inhibitory influences descending from above the spinal cord had been interrupted. This early suggestion of an intrinsic, active inhibition of pain, or at least of the response to a noxious stimulus, would later be seen as having considerable practical and theoretical significance.

The idea that pain has a separate, private pathway in the CNS was supported by research during the last decade of the 19th century and the early 20th century. The development of special tissue stains, a series of animal experiments, and some human postmortem examinations revealed that fibers in the ventrolateral (also called anterolateral) quadrant of the spinal cord ascend above the spinal cord to communicate with a cluster of nerve cells collectively called the *thalamus* (from the Greek "inner chamber";

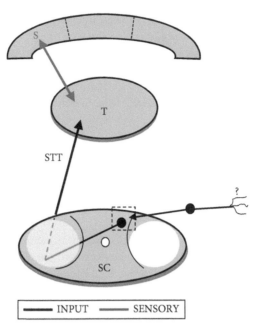

FIGURE 3.1. Diagrammatic representation of the spinothalamic tract (STT) ascending in the white matter of the ventrolateral spinal cord (SC) to the thalamus (T), which is reciprocally connected to the cerebral cortex. STT neuron cell bodies, located in the dorsal gray matter of the opposite side, receive input from sensory neurons with receptor endings in the body or internal organs. The question mark indicates that at the time spinothalamic (aka: ventrolateral or anterolateral) cordotomy was introduced as a treatment for intractable pain, the physiological properties of receptor endings responding to noxious stimulation were unknown.

see Figure A.4 in the Appendix). The thalamus was then known to be the major link between the spinal cord and the cerebral cortex on the brain's surface. The cerebral cortex was also known at the time to be a critical mediator of human sensory experience. The pathway from the ventrolateral spinal cord to the thalamus thus became known as the *spinothalamic tract* (STT; Figure 3.1).

The concept of a spinal cord "pain pathway" gained further support following the 1912 report of clinically significant pain relief after a surgical cut limited to the ventral (anterior) lateral (outside) quadrant of the spinal cord, the location of the STT.[6] Clinical reports with confirmatory autopsies of spinal cord wounds and tumors suggested that lesions within and restricted to this ventrolateral sector of the spinal cord white matter attenuated pain and temperature sensations but left tactile sensations and voluntary motor functions intact. These observations led the neurologist William G. Spiller to suggest that a surgical transection of the ventrolateral spinal cord (ventrolateral cordotomy) would provide one of his patients selective relief from the chronic, severe leg and pelvic pain caused by a tumor near the lower spinal cord.

Before proceeding with the operation, Spiller suggested that two of his surgical colleagues conduct animal experiments to determine if the ventrolateral cordotomy produced a definite loss of evoked pain and if there might be any serious complications of this surgery. Two dogs received a bilateral cordotomy, which was histologically confirmed to be restricted to the ventrolateral spinal cord. Over two months of testing, the investigators found that the withdrawal responses to "extreme heat" and pinching with a hemostat were definitely reduced in both hindlimbs only; in addition, both dogs showed hindlimb clumsiness in walking. The experimenters did not report on the integrity of other cutaneous sensations. Following these results, Dr. Spiller referred his patient to Dr. Edward Martin for bilateral ventrolateral cordotomy (i.e., spinothalamic tractotomy).

Dr. Spiller's patient was a 47-year-old man with a cancerous tumor compressing and perhaps invading the lower spinal cord, causing severe motor and sensory deficits. He complained of severe pain in the pelvis, knees, and ankles and incontinence of urine and stool. He had an almost complete flaccid paralysis, atrophy of both legs, and anesthesia over the buttocks and back of both thighs. Bedside sensory testing revealed a nearly complete loss of touch, deep pinprick, and thermal sensations over the back of each thigh and below the knees; but these sensations were preserved over the anterior thighs and abdomen. His ongoing pain required regular morphine for relief.

On January 19, 1911, Dr. Martin performed a bilateral ventrolateral cordotomy on this patient. The next day, the patient reported a definite and nearly complete relief of his previous ongoing pain and required only a fraction of the previous doses of morphine. Bedside examination 15 months later revealed some reduced pain sensitivity over the anterior thighs but no other sensory changes compared with the preoperative examination. However, the spontaneous, ongoing pain that precipitated the surgery was largely, although incompletely, relieved.

Despite the fact that Dr. Spiller's patient had severe motor and sensory deficits before the surgery and that the consequences of this surgery could not be assessed fully, the clinical case report of Drs. Spiller and Martin became regularly cited as the first successful human ventrolateral cordotomy and heralded the subsequent regular use of this procedure for pain relief over the next eight decades. The apparent clinical utility of spinothalamic tractotomy reinforced the concept of functional localization for pain. Additional support came within the next two decades following the discovery of a group of sensory nerve fibers (discussed in Chapter 6) that produced pain or pain-like responses when electrically stimulated.[7]

Further experience with spinothalamic tractotomy for pain confirms the effectiveness of this procedure for at least temporarily relieving intractable chronic pain while leaving motor and other sensory functions relatively spared; it is especially helpful in relieving pain caused by invasive, incurable cancers. However, very soon after the surgery (often within 24 hours), many patients develop, on the body site opposite the one now rendered analgesic, either a new constant pain or a pain that is evoked by a noxious stimulus applied to the newly analgesic site. This new postoperative pain is sometimes less severe than the original pain but persists among most patients followed for more than a month. The incidence and severity of this problem appears to be correlated with the degree of analgesia produced by the tractotomy; this observation and the rapid onset of the new pain suggest that the STT inhibits a parallel, normally inactive, pathway for pain. In addition, as patients survive longer, it becomes apparent that the operation has additional unwelcome effects probably due to the slow development of persistent anatomical and chemical changes in CNS circuitry (aka: CNS plasticity). Reviews of the results of spinothalamic tractotomy over the ensuing years reveal that, although there is usually a relief of the preoperative pain immediately or soon after the surgery, there is often a return of the original pain or the development of a new pain or unusual, highly unpleasant sensations (called "dysesthesia") in the part of the body rendered hypalgesic by the surgery. These postcordotomy pains or dysesthesias (abnormal sensations) and the return of the original pain can be delayed for months or more than a year, affect up to an estimated 50% or more of long-surviving patients following spinothalamic tractotomy, and cannot be fully explained by differences in surgical procedure or by the return of disease or metastasis of cancer.[8] Rather, these observations show that, following pain-alleviating lesions in the spinal cord, the rostral, brain-directed transmission of impulses leading to pain or other unpleasant experiences can, over time, occur by means other than via the crossed STT. Animal experiments during the last two decades have provided additional information about the neurophysiological mechanisms that may be responsible for these postcordotomy syndromes. Combined behavioral and cellular recording studies show that a thoracic spinothalamic tractotomy on one side causes bursting patterns of neuronal discharges and changes in neuronal responsiveness in the sensory thalamus of both sides. These cellular changes are accompanied by behavioral responses to stimulation that are increased in the hindlimb on the side of the incision and decreased on the opposite side.[9] Dr. Brown-Sequard would be pleased and probably not surprised.

Subsequent clinical observations offer additional evidence that the perception of pain does not depend uniquely or completely on the crossed spinothalamic pathway in the ventrolateral spinal cord.[10] In an attempt to relieve pain on both sides of the body, neurosurgeons began to perform *midline (commissural) myelotomies* to sever the fibers of the STTs of each side where they cross in a commissure in the middle of the spinal cord. The performance of commissural myelotomy led to several remarkable findings that have been independently confirmed by several neurosurgeons and neurologists. First, the pain originating from the clinical condition (usually cancer) can be eliminated even though the patient still feels pain evoked by pinprick, pressure, or heat applied to the hypalgesic or analgesic body area. Some patients report that they feel the stimulus as painful but that the sensation is blunted or muffled; in others, there is no sensory loss detectable by bedside examination even though the pain caused by the disease is absent. Second, the reduction of pain evoked on bedside examination often extends to body areas well above and below the area of analgesia expected by the limited extent of the surgical lesion; in some cases, nearly the entire body is rendered hypalgesic by a very small midline spinal cord incision. Finally, it was later found that a modification of commissural myelotomy relieved pain caused by disease affecting the internal organs (visceral pain) without disturbing other sensory or motor functions. In this "punctate" midline myelotomy, a needle is used to pierce a spot only 5 millimeters into the dorsal (back or posterior) surface of the spinal cord. Animal experiments (rats, monkeys) show that the analgesic effect is due to the interruption of the axons of neuronal cell bodies in the dorsal spinal gray matter.

The clinical and experimental evidence cited previously shows that pain is not completely eliminated after ventrolateral spinal cord lesions and that new painful experiences may appear in the postoperative period. Furthermore, subsequent experience shows that visceral pain can be reduced or eliminated selectively by lesions in dorsal midline parts of the spinal cord, leaving the ventrolateral spinothalamic pathway intact. The presence of pathways for pain parallel to the ventrolateral STT raises the question of the degree to which it has functions that are independent of the integrity of other spinal cord pathways. Does the sensory function of the ventrolateral spinothalamic pathway depend on or interact with other sensory pathways?

To examine this question, a neurophysiologist and a neurosurgeon examined two patients with visually verified lesions (knife wounds) that severed or destroyed most, or in one case all, of the spinal cord except for the ventrolateral quadrant.[11] The result of detailed sensory examinations of these patients up to one and one-half years after injury showed that, as expected, pinprick and temperature stimuli *applied below the lesion* were reliably identified only *opposite* the intact ventrolateral quadrant, consistent with a crossed spinothalamic pain and temperature pathway in the ventrolateral spinal cord. However, in the patient with the most extensive lesion, repetitive pinprick and normally painful hot temperatures applied to the hypalgesic area (on the side of the intact ventrolateral quadrant) evoked "unpleasant" sensations but without the normal sensations of sharpness or heat. Many other neurological clinicians have reported on patients with clinical or otherwise verified STT lesions who experience stimulus-evoked or spontaneous, indescribable, unpleasant sensations on the *same* side of the body as the intact spinal cord and *opposite* the side of the lesion. These observations show that activity in *uncrossed* ascending spinothalamic fibers can lead to the unpleasant (hedonic or affective) aspect of pain but without the information that allows normal sensory identification. Apparently, affective but not normal sensory identification components of the pain experience can be mediated independently via spinal cord pathways other than crossed fibers in the ventrolateral spinal cord[12]; some of these alternate routes will be discussed in Chapter 4.

Spinothalamic tractotomies have been performed also at the level of the brainstem (medulla and midbrain) in an attempt to achieve hypalgesia at the upper torso, shoulder, and head. The problems of incomplete or reappearing pain are similar to those that accompany spinal tractotomies; in addition, the presence of nearby brainstem neural systems essential for respiration and circulatory regulation pose additional risks.

NEUROSURGERY FOR PAIN REVISITED

The limitations of spinothalamic tractotomy prompted attempts to alleviate pain by placing lesions elsewhere, using suction, electocoagulation, or heat coagulation probes inserted into the brain. The choice of targets for focal destruction has been based in large part on what is known about the anatomy of spinothalamic terminations, clinical reports of the effect of cerebral injuries or strokes, and animal experiments. Overall, the results are highly variable and often disappointing because other neurological functions (discussed later) are often disturbed in addition to the variable effects on pain. As with spinothalamic tractotomy, pain sometimes returns, or a new pain or unpleasant dysesthesia appears. The effect of lesions is irreversible and the duration of pain relief, if achieved, is difficult to determine because most of the patients have advanced cancer and die before long-term assessments can be made. Many of the CNS lesion targets are shown in Figure 3.2.

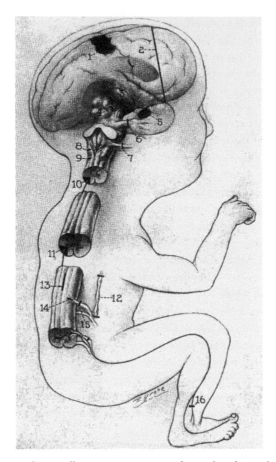

FIGURE 3.2. Schematic diagram illustrating various surgical procedure designed to alleviate pain. 1. Gyrectomy. 2. Prefrontal lobotomy. 3. Thalamotomy. 4. Mesencephalic tractotomy.
5. Hypophysectomy 6. Fifth-nerve rhizotomy. 7. Ninth-nerve neurectomy. 8. Medullary tractotomy.
9. Trigeminal tractotomy. 10. Cervical chordotomy. 11. Thoracic chordotomy. 12. Sympathectomy.
13. Myelotomy. 14. Lissauer tractotomy. 15. Posterior rhizotomy. 16. Neurectomy.
From MacCarty CS, and Drake RL. Neurosurgical procedures for the control of pain. *Proceedings of the Staff
Meetings of the Mayo Clinic 31*: 208–214, 1956. Copyright Elsevier, used with permission.

Lesion locations 4, 8 to 11, 13, and 14 shown in Figure 3.2 are variations on
spinothalamic tractotomy because they are based on what is known about the anatomy
of the STT and the CNS targets of its action potentials. As noted earlier, lesions of purely
sensory nerves in the peripheral nervous system (6, 7, 15, and 16) can be beneficial in
certain conditions but affect other sensory functions such as touch, temperature, and
the sense of movement or limb position. In other words, the denervated part is rendered
anesthetic, not just analgesic or hypalgesic. The use of peripheral neurectomy (16) and
sympathectomy (12) in some chronic pain conditions will be discussed later. But what
has been the rationale for gyrectomy, prefrontal lobotomy, thalamotomy (1 to 3), and
hypophysectomy (5)?

The gyrectomy (removal of all or part of an outfolding of the cerebral cortex) shown in Figure 3.2 refers to the *primary somatic sensory (or S1) cortex*, a brain area known from earlier clinical cases and animal experiments to be critical for tactile sensation. Anatomical studies had shown that this part of the cerebral cortex received axons from a part of the thalamus that in turn received axons from both tactile pathways and from the STT. At the time somatosensory gyrectomies were undertaken, primarily during the 1950s and 1960s, this information suggested the possibility that removing this part of the cortex would relieve chronic, intractable pain in some patients. The possible selective analgesic effect of somatosensory gyrectomy was further suggested by the clinical neurological examination, in the late 1940s and early 1950s, of World War II and some World War I soldiers with bullet wounds of the skull that appeared, on examination at surgery, to damage primarily the S1 cortical area.[13] Some of these patients, when examined months or years following the injury, had reduced or even absent pain and temperature sensation, usually accompanied by impaired tactile sensations, in parts of a hand, arm, or leg; but other patients had exaggerated pain, and still others, with even more extensive cortical lesions, had normal pain and temperature sensation but markedly impaired tactile senses. The neurophysiological basis for these results could not be explained in the absence of postmortem and modern brain imaging studies and remains largely unexplained today. One possibility is that the deep propagation of the force wave from these high-velocity impacts produced subcortical, focal thalamic, or brainstem lesions that were then undetectable.[14] Most S1 neurons respond only to tactile stimuli or joint movement. Contemporary neurophysiological studies of monkeys, however, have revealed a population of neurons in the deep sulcus of S1 cortex that respond differentially or exclusively to noxious stimulation of small areas of the skin and, through their dynamic interactions with neighboring S1 cells, contribute information that is important for perceiving sensory magnitude and the spatiotemporal properties of normal and pathological pain. A detailed mapping of monkey S1 cortex also shows that groups of neurons responding to tactile or to noxious heat stimulation are intermingled throughout anatomical subdivisions of this cortex.[15] Nonetheless, cortical gyrectomy has been largely, if not entirely, abandoned today because of highly variable results, especially for chronic pain, and the usually severe tactile sensory deficits produced by this procedure and by other injuries to S1 and its cortical connections.[16]

Thalamotomy, the placement of lesions in that part of the thalamus that receives spinothalamic input from the spinal cord and brainstem, has been performed on the same rationale as for S1 gyrectomy, again based on the concept that pain has a single, grossly identifiable location in the CNS. Unfortunately, lesions in this part of the thalamus usually impair tactile and other somatosensory functions; moreover, this procedure may produce a *central pain syndrome* in which constant pain is generated within the CNS alone and is perceived as coming from parts of the body opposite the lesion site. Recall the cases especially of Salvatore (but also J.J.), presented in Chapter 1, of examples of pain-related experiences.

Hypophysectomy (removal or destruction of the pituitary gland) was initially used to alleviate pain by reversing or slowing the growth of tissue-invading, endocrine-dependent cancers such as those arising from the prostate or breast. However, the pain relief often occurred long before either endocrine changes or detectable effects on the tumor appeared. Hypophysectomy was also found to be effective for tumors not dependent on endocrine and for pain conditions not caused by cancer. These observations led to the speculation that the *hypothalamus*, which is located just above the pituitary at the base of the brain and regulates the release of pituitary hormones, is somehow involved in alleviating pain. In clinical reports, pain relief is reported to occur without affecting the appreciation of acute pain, pinprick sensitivity, or emotional and cognitive functions; however, there are no studies specifically of these aspects of the operation. Because the mechanism by which hypophysectomy relieves pain is still not known and because of its serious endocrinological consequences, this operation is seldom performed for pain relief today.[17]

The rationale for prefrontal lobotomy and the neurosurgical ablation of other sites outside the known CNS pathways for somatic sensation is based on experiments conducted and theories developed during the latter 19th and early 20th centuries; these are discussed in Chapter 4.

In summary, the attempt to provide a lasting and selective relief from pain by destroying parts of the CNS is disappointing. Early animal experiments show that spinal cord lesions can both decrease and increase responses to noxious stimuli, and subsequent clinical experience shows that pain or other unpleasant sensations often appear later following spinothalamic tractotomy. Accordingly, spinothalamic tractotomy is currently offered primarily to patients with medically intractable pain who are not likely to survive long enough to experience these undesirable postoperative effects. Lesions in other parts of the CNS are often accompanied by the loss of other somatosensory functions and may lead to a central pain syndrome. Furthermore, spinal cord lesions that completely spare the ventrolateral STT are found to produce at least temporary relief of deep visceral pain and, in some cases, total body hypalgesia. Thus, the concept of functional localization of pain in the nervous system is brought into question. There does not appear to be a single, completely private CNS pathway for pain—a structure or pathway that has this function and no other. This raises the question of what is meant by "functional localization." How is function defined? And at what anatomical and structural level is location within the CNS defined? Are there single or multiple points and pathways?

4

EMOTIONS, AFFECT, AND
THE LIMBIC SYSTEM

SHERRINGTON AND PSEUDAFFECTIVE REFLEXES

In 1903, Charles Sherrington (later to become *Sir* Charles Sherrington) conducted a series of observational experiments on dogs whose spinal cords had been completely severed in the cervical (neck) area. He noted that, when a moving tactile or presumably noxious mechanical or thermal stimulus was applied below the spinal lesion, the dog's hind leg, which was paralyzed for voluntary movement, would make several scratches within the stimulated area. This "scratch reflex" was independent of any feeling of itching or need to discard an irritant because there were no connections to the brain; it was organized completely within the spinal cord and depended only on the integrity of the spinal cord and the innervation of the skin.

In subsequent experiments in cats and dogs, both cerebral hemispheres including the thalamus were removed; however, the posterior midbrain (located between the brainstem and thalamus), brainstem, and spinal cord remained intact (see Figure A.4 in the Appendix). In these *decerebrated* animals, a noxious mechanical or thermal stimulus regularly evoked a more elaborate behavioral response that resembled the angry, defensive reaction of a distressed, intact animal. The decerebrated animal would open its eyes with pupils dilated, turn its head toward the stimulated site, bare its teeth, and sometimes snarl and snap. Only noxious stimuli were effective in evoking this response. The full response was brief, lasting only several seconds after the stimulus and followed occasionally by two or three weak head movements or vocalizations within the next minute. Between these evoking stimuli, the animal was quiet and immobile. Because these reflex responses were evoked only by noxious stimuli and fully resembled the reaction of an intact, angry, distressed, and defensive animal to an unpleasant, threatening event, they were called "pseudaffective reflexes." Pseudaffective reflexes required the absence of the cerebral cortex and thalamus but the integrity of the midbrain, brainstem, and certain parts of the spinal cord. Additional experiments revealed that only an intact ventrolateral quadrant of the spinal cord was necessary for the pseudaffective reflex to occur; in fact, the most robust and consistent responses were evoked by noxious stimuli applied to the skin on the side opposite an intact ventrolateral spinal quadrant, indicating that the main pathway crossed within the spinal cord. Thus, Brown-Sequard's observations were confirmed; there was a crossed pathway in the spinal cord that was necessary for these "pain-like" behaviors.[1]

The pseudaffective reflex behaviors did not require most of the brain. However, Sherrington and his colleagues assumed that pain would have been experienced if the brain were intact. They made this assumption because, as the name "pseudaffective" suggests, the behavior they observed conveyed the sense of a negative hedonic or affective experience that is an integral component of pain. They assumed that the reflexive behavior was uncoupled from the experience of pain because the "higher centers" in the thalamus and cerebral cortex were removed and because the evoked behavior was brief and temporally locked to the presence of the noxious stimulus. Accordingly, Sherrington used the phrase "nociceptive reactions" to indicate that the motor signature of pain, the pseudaffective reflex, was triggered by unique "nocicipient" sensory receptors but occurred in the absence of the experience of pain. The nonverbal expression of a feeling state was thus neurophysiologically separated from the feeling itself. Today, the terms "nociceptive" and "nocifensive" are routinely used to refer to animal behaviors that appear to indicate pain but cannot be identified unequivocally as pain in an animal incapable of the linguistic expression of experience.

BARD AND SHAM RAGE

In experiments during the late 1920s, Philip Bard, guided by observations made by Sherrington and others in the late 19th century and early 20th century,[2] showed that removing the cerebral cortex and most of the thalamus of cats produced "sham rage," a behavior that differed from the pseudaffective reflex by being more intense and occurring spontaneously or following mild tactile stimuli or gentle movement.[3] Noxious stimulation of the skin, however, was most effective in evoking this behavior consistently. In sham rage, the animal would suddenly bare its teeth, snarl, make biting movements, and assume a posture of attack or defense. The pupils would dilate, fur would become erect, and sweat would appear on the toe pads as evidence that the sympathetic (norepinephrine) component of the autonomic peripheral nervous system (aPNS) had become activated (see the Appendix) as part of an overall mechanism for defending against injury. Between outbursts of this rage-like behavior, the animals were quiet, presumably because they lacked a sustained feeling of the fear and rage suggested by their behavior—hence the term "sham rage." By carefully adjusting the extent of brain destruction, Bard showed that the integrity of the *hypothalamus* (just below the thalamus and above the pituitary (see Figure A.4 in the Appendix) and the most caudal (posterior) and ventral parts of the thalamus was necessary for the full expression of this behavior. Thus, the experiments of Bard and Sherrington and their colleagues showed that the behavioral and autonomic expression of physical defense was tightly coupled to noxious stimulation. The behavior resembled that associated with intensely negative affective experiences, but the neural mechanisms necessary to actually feel pain were missing, lying somewhere within the thalamus and cortex of the brain that had been excised and discarded.

PAPEZ AND THE EMOTIONAL BRAIN

So what neural structures lead from "nociception" and "nociceptive behavior" to pain? What circuitry gives nociception the affective dimension that makes it painful? Nearly a decade after Bard's observations, James W. Papez, then a neuroanatomist at Cornell, wrote the following:

It is proposed that the hypothalamus, the anterior thalamic nuclei, the gyrus cinguli, the hippocampus and their interconnections constitute a harmonious mechanism which may elaborate the functions of central emotion, as well as participate in emotional expression.[4]

In formulating his hypothesis, Papez focused on the hypothalamus (see *p* and *t*, Figure 4.1) as the key structure shown by Bard to be critical for generating the somatic and autonomic expression of emotional behavior. Papez used a combination of neuroanatomical, neurophysiological, and clinical information to marshal evidence that the hypothalamus, acting through connected structures in the temporal lobe and thalamus, could excite neurons of the cingulate gyrus in the medial wall of each cerebral hemisphere (see *gc* in Figure 4.1). Based on the available (and at the time sparse) clinical evidence that damage to the cingulate cortex resulted in apathy, indifference, loss of emotional spontaneity, and varying degrees of somnolence, he then declared that "the cingular

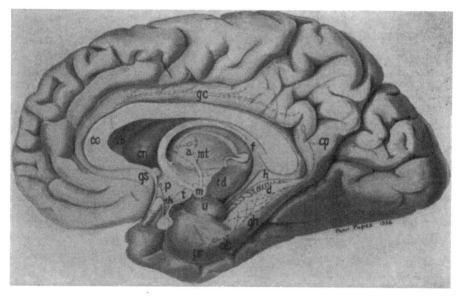

FIGURE 4.1. Medial (inside) surface of the right hemisphere, showing the brain structures postulated by Papez to constitute the neural basis for affective (hedonic) experiences. Frontal lobe is to the left, occipital lobe to the right. The *thalamus* is the large, round structure in the middle, just below the corpus callosum (*cc*), and the label "a" refers to an anterior (frontal) cluster (nucleus) of thalamic neurons that are reciprocally connected with the cingulate gyrus. The pituitary gland can be seen hanging like a bell just below the *hypothalamus*; the letters "p" and "t" refer to parts of the hypothalamus. The caudate nucleus (*cn*), a component of the *basal ganglia* (discussed later), can be seen anterior to (in front of) the thalamus. *a*, Anterior nucleus (of the thalamus); *ab*, angular bundle; *cn*, caudate nucleus; *cc*, corpus callosum; *cp*, cingulum posterius; *d*, gyrus dentatus; *f*, fornix; *gc*, gyrus cinguli; *gh*, gyrus hippocampi; *gs*, gyrus subcallosus; *h*, hippocampus nudus; *m*, mamillary body; *mt*, mamillothalamic tract; *p*, pars óptica hypothalamic; *pr*, pyriform area; *sb*, subcallosal bundle; *f*, tuber cinereum; *td*, tractus mamillotegmentalis; *th*, tractus hypophyseus; *u*, uncus.

From Papez JW. A proposed mechanism of emotion. *Archives of Neurological Psychiatry* 38: 725–743, 1937, with permission from the American Medical Association.

[or cingulate] gyrus may be looked on as the receptive region for the experiencing of emotion as the result of impulses coming from the hypothalamic region. . . ."[5] Thus, the hypothalamus, a tiny but critical structure at the base of the brain, and the cingulate cortex, along the lower medial wall of each hemisphere, became the proposed centers for the downstream expression and upstream experience of affective feeling and emotion. Although Papez did not express it, an obvious conclusion would have been that the decorticate and decerebrate animals studied by Sherrington, Bard, and others would have actually experienced pain and possibly rage if the circuitry he described, especially the hypothalamus and cingulate gyrus, had been intact. In the decade following Papez's proposal, the cingulate cortex, hypothalamus, parts of the thalamus, nearby subcortical basal ganglia, and temporal lobe were conceptually united as the "limbic system,"[6] a reference to the fact that the cingulate gyrus and medial temporal lobe form a border (limbus) around the upper brainstem. Subsequent research confirms and refines the concept that at least some of the structures comprising the limbic system and anatomically related structures are critical participants in the generation of autonomic functions and both positive and negative hedonic states.[7]

PAIN: A SYNTHETIC EXPERIENCE AND A NEW CONCEPTUAL MODEL

Because pseudaffective and sham rage behaviors are most effectively evoked by noxious stimuli and depend on a crossed spinal pathway from the ventrolateral spinal cord, the Papez circuit for emotion and affect is functionally associated with the spinothalamic tract (STT) and, therefore, with pain. But what circuitry establishes this relationship? A critical anatomical link connecting the STT and the limbic system comes from studies during the late 1950s and early 1960s; these show that, in monkeys and humans, ventrolateral spinal cord axons send synaptic terminals directly into both *outer (lateral) and inner (medial) parts of the thalamus* and into the *reticular formation (RF) of the brainstem* at several levels between the spinal cord and thalamus[8] (Figure 4.2).

The thalamus (from the Greek *thalamos*, meaning "inner chamber")[9] is composed of groups of subcortical neurons (see Figure A.4 in the Appendix) that receive sensory information and communicate reciprocally with the overlying cerebral cortex. The *outer* or *lateral* part of the thalamus receives part of the direct STT endings and transmits information to the primary (S1) and secondary (S2) somatosensory cortices as well as to nearby cortical areas (including the insula, which will be discussed later). Neurons within the primary thalamocortical somatosensory pathway respond to stimulation of small areas of the body (e.g., part of a finger or limb), and the intensity of their response often correlates with the intensity of the stimulus; a few respond primarily to noxious stimuli. Destructive lesions within the thalamocortical (primarily S1) neuronal system greatly impair somatic sensory discriminative functions such as identifying, through exploration, the presence, location, or movement of an object on the skin; sometimes, the sense of limb position or the shape or sharpness of an object is affected also. Overall, this outer or lateral part of the thalamus and its cortical connection is physiologically suited to encode information about stimulus location, duration, movement, and intensity.[10] By contrast, neurons within the *inner or medial* thalamus often respond to some

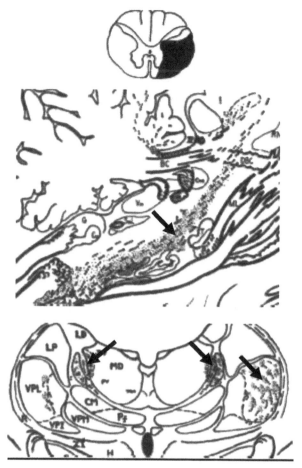

FIGURE 4.2. Some direct connections of axons (*small dots and stipple*) in the ventrolateral spinal cord (*top*) with the reticular formation of the brainstem (*middle, arrow*) and thalamus (*bottom; me-dial and intralaminar [double arrows] and ventral posterolateral [single arrow]*).

Adapted from Mehler WR, Feferman ME, and Nauta WJH. Ascending axon degeneration following antero-lateral cordotomy: An experimental study in the monkey. *Brain 83*: 718–750, 1960, with permission of Oxford University Press.

combination of innocuous or noxious stimuli but are excited by stimuli applied any-where within a large area (e.g., half or all of the body); in addition, their responses usu-ally show poorer correlations with spatial, temporal, and intensive stimulus properties.[11] In humans, the relatively rare destructive lesions confined within this territory do not impair somatosensory discriminative functions; rather, they are associated with cog-nitive deficits including memory loss, affective indifference, and emotional blunting.[12] Most important, many midline, medial, and intralaminar thalamic neurons have strong connections to limbic system structures and consequently have been referred to as the "limbic thalamus."[13] It is by way of these inner thalamic neurons and their brainstem connections that spinothalamic fibers ascending in the ventrolateral spinal cord gain ac-cess to the autonomic and hedonic functions of the limbic system.

But there is an additional pathway that connects the somatosensory and limbic systems. The RF is a phylogenetically ancient neuronal system that forms the interior core of the *brainstem* between the spinal cord and the thalamus; it contains a complex network of neurons with extensive connections to both the thalamus, hypothalamus, several subcortical brain structures (e.g., basal ganglia), and the spinal cord. Neurophysiological and anatomical experiments in the mid-20th century showed that parts of the RF are essential for maintaining the brain in wakefulness and that it receives somatic and visceral sensory input that is transmitted to thalamic neurons connected to subcortical and cortical components of the limbic system (i.e., the *limbic thalamus*). These ascending connections to the brain reside within the core of the brainstem at several levels above the spinal cord and do not depend on intact direct STT connections.[14] Sensory input to the reticular formation comes from neurons within the spinal cord gray matter. Some of these spinal cord cells discharge most rapidly during noxious stimulation, and many RF cells show similar nociceptive responses. The participation of the RF in pain-related behaviors is indicated further by the observation that electrical stimulation within parts of the RF triggers or facilitates aversive escape behaviors, while destructive focal lesions reduce them. However, in addition to the connections ascending to the brain, many brainstem RF neurons send axons to sensory and motor neurons in the spinal cord. Recordings from awake animals show that many RF neurons are active during specific movements, including some employed during aversive escape. One heuristic suggestion is that the RF uses information from sensory receptors and other central nervous system (CNS) structures to organize patterns of muscular activity into complex behaviors, including, but not limited to, those related to the detection or threat of injury. This conjecture is consistent with the observed pseudaffective and sham rage behaviors of decerebrate and decorticate animals discussed previously. Although the complex and heterogeneous properties of the RF make it difficult, if not impossible, to offer a fully unifying summary of RF function, it nonetheless seems reasonable to conclude that the brainstem RF provides a route, in parallel with the direct STT, for the transmission and distribution of behaviorally significant nociceptive information to the spinal cord, to the thalamus, and to limbic structures of the brain.[15]

Based on the previous considerations alone, pain could be conceived of as a hedonically negative somatic sensory experience mediated by at least two anatomically and functionally distinct but interacting neural circuits: one, the somatosensory network of the lateral thalamus and parietal cortex that codes for sensory qualities (e.g., timing, location, intensity, and receptor source); and another, represented by spinothalamic and brainstem connections with the limbic system, that codes for the aversive, unpleasant, hedonic quality of pain. This formulation is consistent with the concept of the CNS organized as a parallel distributed processing system.[16] According to this model, "pain" is a label for an experience synthesized by the conjoint activity of these physiologically distinct neuronal systems. *Pain does not exist independent of this synthesis.*[17]

Of course, every sensation or experience is a synthesis. The CNS receives information from a wide variety of sensors, some with very limited and some with a broad range of sensitivities to physical events in the environment. The human CNS integrates this information to develop unique subjective experiences and behaviors. The type of synthesis proposed in the conceptual model referenced here is derived by decomposing the experience of pain into three dimensions: discriminative, motivational or affective, and cognitive, each of which is a lower level synthesis developed by distinct but interacting neural circuits. Pain results from the synthesis of limbic (hedonic), somatosensory (discriminative), and integrative frontoparietal cortical (cognitive) neuronal activity. Pain emerges only *during the conjoint activity* of limbic and somatosensory systems, thus allowing discriminative (sensory) and hedonic (affective) features to be perceived as components of pain as modified by high-order (cognitive) processes. Thus, the behavioral effect of neuronal responses to noxious stimulation depends on close connections with other groups of neurons. Neurons responding to a noxious heat stimulus may, depending on their immediate connectivity, contribute to the perception of changes in heat intensity, to defensive posturing, to changes in autonomic activity, to the hedonic component of pain, or to some combination of these. For example, some neurons within the primary (S1) somatosensory parietal cortex respond preferentially to noxious stimuli, but because of their immediate connectivity, their destruction results in a loss of stimulus recognition or detection—not to affective or cognitive blunting, nor to a specific impairment of movement.[18]

The merging of sensation and affect was later incorporated into a definition of pain adopted by the IASP[19]: "An unpleasant sensory and emotional experience associated with actual or potential tissue damage, or described in terms of such damage." That pain emerges from the coactivation of hedonically neutral (sensory) and hedonically weighted (affective) mechanisms was soon explicitly recognized by the development and subsequent widespread clinical application of the McGill Pain Questionnaire and pain rating scales that separately measure these components of the pain experience.[20]

Meanwhile, back in the operating room, the association of the limbic system with pain provided the rationale for surgical ablative procedures directed at the frontal lobe, particularly the anterior cingulate cortex. Perhaps the hedonic or affective component of medically intractable pain could be relieved while avoiding the complications and limitations of spinothalamic tractotomy. For that matter, why not ablate portions of the cingulate gyrus to relieve the hedonic burden of a variety of psychiatric disorders? As documented in a recent review of this topic, surgical ablations within the cingulate cortex have been, and continue to be, performed for both psychiatric disorders and chronic, intractable pain.[21] The results are quite variable, but even when the target condition is reported to have been at least partially relieved, the reports indicate that patients are left with some impairments of attention, behavioral spontaneity, and executive function. Consequently, this procedure has a very limited application, usually for only the most severely affected or terminally ill patients.

To summarize some of the major concepts prevailing at the time of the Issaquah meeting, I have constructed the diagram in Figure 4.3. We knew that there were physiologically specialized receptors in the skin, and presumably in subcutaneous and visceral structures also, that responded primarily or exclusively to noxious stimuli or to the consequences of tissue damage. (The question mark near the peripheral nerve endings of Figure 3.1 has been removed.) We knew that these nociceptors generated action potentials in small-diameter peripheral sensory nerves that excited STT neurons in the dorsal gray matter (*dashed box*, Figure 4.3) of the spinal cord. At the time of the Issaquah meeting, neurophysiological studies of STT neurons had just begun. Nearly

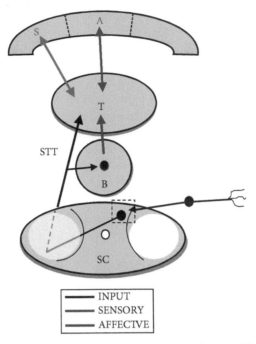

FIGURE 4.3. Conceptual model of pain mechanisms prevailing at the time of the Issaquah meeting. Abbreviations as in Figure 3.1 plus: S, sensory-discriminative functions of somatosensory cortex; A, affective functions of limbic system cortical areas; B, brain stem connections to thalamic neurons.

seven years earlier, recordings from cat spinal cord sensory axons revealed that many of them responded to electrical stimuli that excited both myelinated A and unmyelinated C fibers and that repetitions of those stimuli produced progressively prolonged responses (later called "windup") of these neurons. The proposed mechanism underlying this C fiber–enhanced response supported the "gate control" theory of pain.[22]

Within a year of the Issaquah meeting, recordings of action potentials from monkey spinal cord STT neurons revealed that some of them responded only to noxious stimulation of the skin (later called "nociceptive-specific" or NS neurons), while others responded to both noxious and innocuous stimuli (later called "wide dynamic range" or WDR neurons).[23] The coexistence of WDR and NS neurons generated an ongoing and often heated debate about which of these types of neurons is responsible for pain. The major argument for NS cells is that their response best reflects the clear distinction between painful and painless. The argument for WDR cells is that, even if the painful-painless distinction has a clear threshold and is always unambiguous (which it is not), a clear distinction between painful and painless does not require that neurons remain silent before engaging the brain mechanisms necessary for pain. Think of filling a glass with water, with the water level representing action potential frequency. When the water level just exceeds the top of the glass, an obvious threshold event occurs; painless (everything before the spill) becomes painful (the spill). The NS versus WDR argument continues among those whom, for whatever reasons, feel forced to choose between them.

However, it is possible, even likely, that both types of neurons contribute to the distinction between painless and painful.[24]

At the time, we knew that physiologically specialized neurons in the thalamus (T in Figure 4.2) received STT input and transmitted nociceptive information to somatic sensory neurons (S in Figure 4.2) in the parietal lobe of the cerebral cortex, enabling the identification of the spatial, temporal, and intensive features of the stimulus. And we knew that nociceptive activation of the STT was tightly linked to negatively hedonic or affective behavioral responses and, in humans, to experiences mediated through RF neurons in the upper brainstem (*arrow*, B), hypothalamus, thalamus, and affective circuitry (A) in the cerebral cortex and associated limbic system structures. But we also knew that the experience of pain could be modified and could vary considerably among individuals and even within the same individual. In everyday life and in some extraordinary circumstances (see earlier section on sample of pain experiences), the stimulation of nociceptors does not always result in pain, and pain intensity does not always correlate with the degree of tissue damage or other measures of nociceptor activity. Although we understood that brain activity, including attention and cognitive functions, profoundly affects pain,[25] we were then just beginning to learn about the neural mechanisms underlying this modulating effect.

5

EARLY EVIDENCE OF CENTRAL NERVOUS SYSTEM CONTROL AND A CONCEPTUAL MODEL REVISITED

The concept that brain activity is a major determinant of sensory experience has been around for a long time. In his 1949 book, *The Organization of Behavior*, D. O. Hebb[1] briefly reviewed the history of this idea, contrasting it with the concept that sensory experience is determined almost exclusively by sensory receptors. Citing evidence then available, Hebb wrote: "[behavioral] responses are determined by something else besides the immediately preceding sensory stimulation. [This] does not deny the importance of the immediate stimulus; it does deny that sensory stimulation is everything in behavior."[2] He went on to give examples of attention, past experience, expectation, and other central processes as critical determinants of perception and sensory experience generally. Subsequent research and clinical observation, as discussed later, have amply verified this view for many sensory experiences, including pain.

ANATOMY

One obvious indication that the brain must have a powerful effect on somatic sensory experience is simply the anatomy of the central nervous system (CNS). The human brain (cerebral cortex, thalamus, and basal ganglia; see Figure A.4 in the Appendix) comprises 85% of the total volume of the CNS, while the cerebellum takes up 10%, and the brainstem and spinal cord occupy only 5% (Figure 5.1). Because the direction and dominance of information flow within the CNS is likely to be related to the number of axons within a pathway, it is important to note that, at the rostral (highest or upper) level of the human spinal cord, the number of axons *ascending* in the spinothalamic tract (STT) of one side is estimated to be in the range of several thousand, whereas, at a similar anatomical level, the number of axons *descending* directly from the cerebral cortex to the spinal cord is estimated to be more than one million. These *corticospinal* axons terminate in the ventral spinal gray matter among motor neurons that innervate voluntary muscles but also among sensory neurons at the origin of the STT in the dorsal spinal cord gray matter. Farther upstream at the level of the thalamus, where STT axons terminate, nearly half of all synapses on thalamic neurons sending axons to the cerebral cortex come from the cortex itself.[3]

Of course, comparative volume alone does not tell us much about functional relationships. The hypothalamus, for example, is a tiny neural structure with functions that are essential for many vital bodily functions, including, as discussed in the Appendix, actions of the autonomic peripheral nervous system (PNS), temperature and osmotic control,

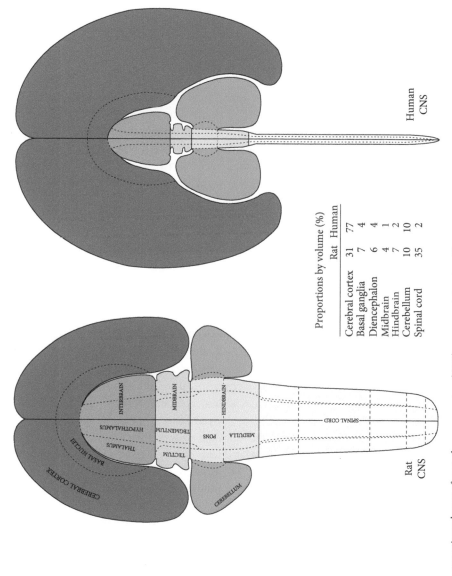

Proportions by volume (%)		
	Rat	Human
Cerebral cortex	31	77
Basal ganglia	7	4
Diencephalon	6	4
Midbrain	4	1
Hindbrain	7	2
Cerebellum	10	10
Spinal cord	35	2

FIGURE 5.1. Comparative volumes of central nervous system (CNS) components in rat and human.

From Swanson LW. Mapping the human brain: Past, present, and future. *Trends in Neurosciences 18: 471–474*, 1995, with permission from Elsevier.

hormonal balance, and affective behaviors. Nonetheless, even considering counting errors, the numerical difference between direct ascending and descending axonal pathways is impressive and consistent with an important "top-down" influence of brain activity on sensory experience. This comparison does not include indirect connections through which cortical actions may be transmitted to the spinal cord through relays in the brainstem. Based on an inspection of this anatomical arrangement, an extraterrestrial visitor could reasonably conclude that brains, especially those of humans, evolved primarily as exploratory organs that are informed, but not predominantly driven, by sensory information transmitted via the spinal cord.

NEUROPHYSIOLOGY

In 1954 and 1959, two neurophysiological experiments showed that electrical stimulation of various CNS structures and pathways decreases or increases the stimulus-evoked and spontaneous activity of somatic sensory neurons in the spinal cord.[4] This "centrifugal" effect was demonstrated by electrical stimulation within the cerebellum, the somatic sensory areas of the cerebral cortex, the cingulate gyrus of the limbic system, and the reticular formation of the brainstem. There was evidence that these centrifugal CNS influences are present in the absence of stimulation, can be eliminated by general anesthesia, and provide an essential, ongoing (or "tonic") background for the transmission of sensory information.

Within the next decade, additional experiments provided neuroanatomical and neurophysiological evidence that brain and brainstem mechanisms exerted a controlling influence on somatic and visceral sensory inputs. In the anesthetized cat, some thalamic neurons were found to respond only to noxious cutaneous stimuli; however, in the awake monkey, nociceptive thalamic responses were shown to vary with the level of behavioral arousal. In an especially dramatic demonstration of CNS control, continuous electrical current applied within the upper brainstem of awake rats eliminated any evidence of pain (including that of abdominal surgery) without obviously affecting motor function or other behaviors. These experiments give physiological and functional significance to the anatomical dominance of the brain and brainstem, especially in modulating pain.[5] Subsequent research, to be considered later, reveals some of the neurophysiological mechanisms that mediate this modulation of noxious sensory information.

One obvious way of modifying pain-related sensory information is by direct excitation or, through interneurons, inhibition of STT neurons in the spinal cord gray matter. In 1974 and for several years thereafter, experiments showed that electrical stimulation in the brainstem or cerebral cortex could both excite and inhibit spinal cord STT neurons.[6] The direct excitation or inhibition of STT neurons tends to affect their responses to PNS inputs from both tactile and nociceptive sensory fibers (see the Appendix for more discussion of the somatic and autonomic PNS). But a more selective way of modulating sensory responses is to control the synaptic effectiveness of some inputs while leaving others either unaffected or responsive to other stimuli. As noted in the Appendix, the amount of neurotransmitter released by a presynaptic ending is affected by the presynaptic membrane potential, which in turn affects calcium channels that mobilize presynaptic vesicles containing a neurotransmitter. In the dorsal gray matter of the spinal cord (see *dashed box* in Figure 4.3), there are small, short-axoned neurons (*interneurons*), some of which have presynaptic endings on the presynaptic endings of sensory fibers entering the spinal cord (a synapse on a synapse). Some of these interneurons release gamma-aminobutyric acid (GABA), a neurotransmitter that activates receptors on the presynaptic membrane and reduces the presynaptic release of an excitatory neurotransmitter either by depolarization (primary afferent depolarization, or PAD) or by directly reducing the presynaptic calcium currents that mediate the neurotransmitter release.[7] Other neurotransmitters, such as norepinephrine, serotonin, or opiate-like peptides, have similar modulating effects on spinal sensory neurons either through synaptic (axo-axonal) mechanisms or simply by their presence in the surrounding extracellular space. The interneurons that affect spinal sensory cells receive synaptic input from a variety of sources, including the cerebral cortex of the CNS and sensory fibers from the PNS.

Some of the earliest neurophysiological studies of spinal cord sensory input revealed the depolarizing (inhibitory) effects of one group of sensory fibers on another. An important component of the gate control hypothesis included a combination of PAD and presynaptic *hyper*polarization (PAH), which could selectively increase the excitatory effect of some sensory inputs and decrease that of others, thereby expanding the opportunities for selectively controlling the transmission of sensory information at the spinal cord level. Some of the subsequent research suggested that stimulation of relatively thick, large-diameter, touch-sensitive "A" nerve fibers could possibly attenuate the pain evoked by activity in the thin, small-diameter nociceptive "A-delta" and "C" fibers through PAD mechanisms within the spinal cord, but the neurophysiology continues to be investigated. The predicted pain-modulating effect of electrically stimulating tactile-sensitive PNS nerve fibers led to the commercial development of transcutaneous nerve stimulation (TENS) devices that are still used today for localized pain relief in some patients.[8] The presynaptic inhibition of one set of sensory fibers by another is one possible explanation for why scratching, rubbing, or even other noxious stimuli can partially relieve pain or itching.

NEUROPHARMACOLOGY

Finally, at the time of the Issaquah meeting, membrane-bound receptors for opiate (morphine-like) compounds had just been identified in the mammalian CNS, and within the next three years, an opiate-like (opioid) compound was found in the mammalian brain where opiate receptors are also located. Opioid receptors were also found on the endings of PNS sensory fibers within the dorsal gray matter of the primate spinal cord.[9] These findings give added significance to the known neurophysiology of sensory control by showing that analgesic drugs such as morphine and its derivatives activate these built-in, endogenous mechanisms directly through drug-specific receptors in the CNS. The evolutionary process has apparently retained selected elements of the plant world, including the marijuana component of hemp, by providing receptors for their hypalgesic and psychic effects in mammalian brains.[10]

Figure 5.2 is a *final diagrammatic summary* of the information about pain mechanisms that was available at the time of the Issaquah meeting. The major differences from Figure 4.3 include the addition of descending influences from the brain (*curved arrows*)

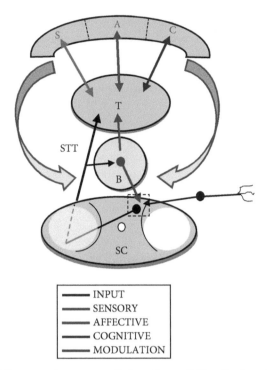

FIGURE 5.2. Final diagrammatic summary of information available at the time of the Issaquah meeting, emphasizing the emerging evidence for "top-down" central controls from the brain stem (B) and from interacting sensory (S), affective (A), and cognitive (C) mechanisms in the cerebral cortex. These descending pathways modulate the excitability of spinothalamic tract neurons in the dorsal gray matter the spinal cord (dashed box).

and brainstem (*straight arrow* from B), and the addition of arrows depicting the interaction among sensory (S), affective (A), and cognitive (C) functions of the cerebral cortex and associated limbic system structures. Overall, the figure depicts a conceptual model in which information about actual or potential tissue injury is widely distributed among functionally distinct CNS structures that, in turn, modulate this information at several different levels of information transmission. This is not to suggest that this conceptual model was embraced or even contemplated by most of the attendees at the Issaquah meeting, but the informational framework for the model depicted here was available then, in the mid-1970s.

PROGRESS SINCE THE ISSAQUAH MEETING

An advanced, focused Ovid Medline search for all archived articles with "pain" (unrestricted language) in the title, abstract, subject heading, or as a keyword for the 41 years from 1974 to 2015 yields 436,849 articles, an annual publication rate of 10,655 articles. The same search for the 41 years *before* 1973 (since 1932) brings up 15,913 articles, or approximately 388 articles per year. Thus, the annual publication rate for "pain" articles has increased almost 30-fold in the comparable period of time since the Issaquah meeting. (By comparison, the world population increased 82.5% during this period.) Of course, this crude analysis includes all Medline "pain" articles regardless of their relevance to basic or applied pain research or medical practice. Also, a comparable increase in publication rate has almost certainly occurred in most other scholarly disciplines. Nonetheless, the numbers reveal a dramatic increase in pain-related publications since the formation of the International Association for the Study of Pain.

Mogil and colleagues conducted a far more sophisticated analysis of publications in the journal *Pain* from its inception in 1975 through 2007, showing an approximate 50-fold increase in published papers over this 32-year period. The authors specifically noted that, during this period, there was an increase in the percentage of pharmacological studies using animal models of pain behavior but a marked decrease in the proportion of reports on pain interventions, such as clinical trials, in humans.[11] The reasons for this shift in content are unexplained but include the possibility that the clinical application of treatments suggested by animal models (aka: translational research) is more difficult than anticipated.

It is not surprising that much has happened since the meeting in Issaquah. As in other areas of research, there has been an outpouring of information during the past four decades that has, in effect, overwhelmed the comprehensive capacity of individuals, research groups, and entire institutions. Any attempt to present this information in any detail would be foolhardy in the extreme. Here, I will offer a highly distilled synthesis of a mountain of data and the basic concepts emerging from them. I have focused on a few areas in which new information might be expected to have an impact on clinical practice, patient care, and our understanding of nervous system function generally.

6

PSYCHOPHYSICS AND NOCICEPTORS

PSYCHOPHYSICS

What is a nociceptor? One definition could be that a nociceptor is a tissue-resident structure that triggers action potentials in its attached nerve fiber only during a normally painful stimulus. As will be apparent from the following discussion, that definition is at best incomplete and at least misleading. Recall that, in the early 20th century, Sir Charles Sherrington inferred the existence of specialized nociceptors based on the physical characteristics of the somatic stimulus that reliably elicited pseudaffective reflexes or more elaborate behavior in spinalized and decerebrate dogs and cats. It was the animal's behavior that led to this inference. When the electrophysiological recording of action potentials from single sensory axons became possible about a half-century later, the existence of a nociceptor was likewise inferred from the physical properties of the stimulus—on the assumption, however reasonable, that the stimulus would be perceived as painful by a fully sentient animal. Of course, the only sentient animal capable of providing a reliable and fully descriptive account of its experience is a human. Therefore, to fully define "nociceptor," it was necessary to link human reports to some measurement of action potential activity in sensory fibers of the peripheral nervous system (PNS).

Action potentials (aka: spikes) generated by a single neuron all have the same amplitude (in millivolts; see the Appendix), so neuronal responses, including the activity of single sensory fibers, are quantified by some measure of spike activity, such as frequency (e.g., spikes/second, interspike interval). The measurement of human responses or descriptions of sensory experience is more complicated but is nonetheless used regularly in medical practice (think of audiograms or eye charts). The field of *psychophysics* developed to enable investigators to quantify various aspects of human sensory experience (e.g., intensity, color, pitch, pleasantness, unpleasantness) by briefly training people to report their experience on a numerical scale (e.g., 0 to 10) in relation to some physical property of the stimulus (pressure, temperature, wavelength, chemical concentration). Psychophysical studies of somatic sensations, for example, show that it is possible to determine a quantitative relationship between changes in the application of a stimulus (e.g., thermal, mechanical) and changes in the perception of intensity, duration, and, in the case of pain, the hedonic component of unpleasantness. It is important to realize that, when asking a person to rate "pain" on a single scale, the response will be determined by both the sensory (discriminative and affectively neutral) and hedonic (aversive, unpleasant) components of the experience.[1] Psychophysics is a critically important part of pain research because it allows researchers to relate measures of subjective experience to neuronal activity.[2]

Perhaps the simplest form of psychophysics is the determination of threshold, the stimulus intensity necessary for simple detection or for detecting differences in stimulus intensity (discrimination threshold). There is a long history of attempts to determine a "pain threshold" in humans, but the contemporary era began in the mid to late 20th century with the development of methods to deliver controlled thermal and mechanical stimuli to human skin. The results show that, under controlled laboratory conditions, it is possible to determine thresholds for pain induced by heat, cold, mechanical, and chemical stimulation. Heat stimulation has the advantage of being relatively easy to standardize and apply across different populations of humans and animals, thus accounting for the predominance of heat pain studies in the pain research literature. Thresholds and other measures of pain can also be obtained for cold, mechanical, and chemical stimuli, but they are generally more difficult to standardize and apply in different laboratory and clinical settings.

For technical reasons, the most practical, reliable, and frequently used method is to apply heat with a stimulator in contact with the skin; this also has the advantage of resembling the way we usually experience heat pain—by contacting a hot object. Figure 6.1 is a histogram showing the distribution of 326 people of both sexes in the 20- to 30-year age range who identified a contact heat stimulus as moderately painful when applied to the hairless undersurface of the forearm for 10 seconds; the average temperature required to elicit this response was 44.1° C (about 111° F). These results for the arm are very similar to those obtained earlier in a separate laboratory in a population of 32 healthy persons; the threshold averaged 45.6° C for "moderate" pain and

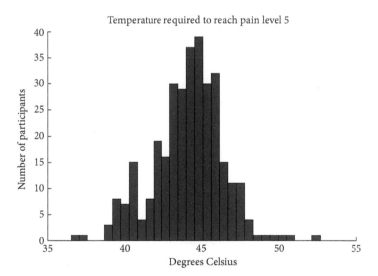

FIGURE 6.1. This histogram shows the distribution of 326 people of both sexes in the 20- to 30-year age range, who identified different contact heat temperatures as moderately painful ("level 5" in the figure title) when applied to the hairless undersurface of the forearm for 10 seconds. The average temperature that was required to elicit this response was 44.1° C (about 111° F). On the rating scale used here, level 2 is just barely painful, and level 8 is near the limit of tolerance.
Data courtesy of Professor Tor D. Wager, Department of Psychology, University of Colorado, Boulder.

44.6° C for "slight" pain, but the stimulus duration was about 4 seconds instead of 10.[3] These results have been confirmed in many other studies and suggest that a nociceptor in the relatively hairless skin of the forearm, if it responds to heat at all, should either become active (generate action potentials) at approximately 45° C or show a marked increase in activity at or near this temperature. Heat pain thresholds and other pain intensity measures have been determined for other body sites such as the palms, soles, and face. There is modest site-related variation, but it is nonetheless possible to obtain data that relate pain systematically across populations to some heat stimulus parameter like intensity, duration, or some combination of the two.

NOCICEPTORS AND THEIR FIBERS

Recordings from the cutaneous nerves of cats, rats, monkeys, and humans show that putative cutaneous nociceptors generate action potentials in the thinnest fibers within nerves of the PNS.[4] These fibers fall into two groups. Each fiber of one group, called *A-delta* fibers (for historical reasons irrelevant for this story) is wrapped along its length by a thin layer of non-neural cells (glia) that form a coating called myelin; the other and thinnest group, called *C* fibers (nomenclature again irrelevant for now), has no myelin coating (i.e., they are unmyelinated fibers). Because of biophysical properties provided by their myelin coatings, A-delta fibers conduct their action potentials much more rapidly than C fibers (on average, between 15 and 20 compared with approximately 2 to 0.5 meters/second), but some fibers in both groups are most active (show fastest spiking) during heat, mechanical, or chemical stimuli that could be reasonably considered noxious. (By contrast, a third group of thickly myelinated fibers [called *A-beta*] have action potential conduction velocities of 60 or more meters/second and respond only to light tactile stimulation, muscle stretching, or joint movement.)

There are two classes of nociceptive C fibers based on their embryonic history, biochemical characteristics, and connections within the upper layers of the dorsal gray matter of the mammalian spinal cord. One group is called "peptidergic" because it contains specific peptides that can function as neurotransmitters; their pharmacological ablation in mice almost eliminates behavioral responses to noxious heat, but not to noxious cold or mechanical stimulation. The other group, non–peptidergic C nociceptors, appears to be necessary to maintain the responsiveness of mice to noxious mechanical, but not heat stimulation. However, when both groups of C fibers are eliminated or at least greatly reduced in number, mice continue to display full but slightly delayed pain-related behavior during inflammation induced by the subcutaneous injection of formalin. These rodent experiments reveal some of the biological and functional diversity within the group of nociceptive C fibers and also suggest that the lightly myelinated A-delta fibers can maintain some nociceptive functions in the absence of C fiber activity.[5] The significance of these observations for humans and clinical pain conditions remains to be determined.

It is important to note that some C or A-delta sensory fibers do not have nociceptors for sensory endings; in fact, many respond primarily or exclusively to innocuous thermal or mechanical stimulation. The exact proportion of non-nociceptive C and A-delta fibers is not known, but some researchers have estimated that as many as 70% of the C fiber population innervating the hairy skin of the human forearm show maximum responses to gentle tactile stimulation, often requiring several seconds of slowly moving contact with the skin. The location of these fibers on hairy skin, their preferential responses to slow stroking stimuli, and the recent evidence that their activity is associated with pleasant tactile sensations and excitation of the cerebral cortex have prompted the speculation that they contribute to the hedonically positive (erotic?) aspects of touch. In addition, a significant population of C fibers respond only to innocuous thermal stimuli, primarily warmth, and are likely to contribute to basic thermoregulatory functions. Some A-delta fibers also respond primarily or exclusively to brief, innocuous tactile or thermal stimulation. Because of the high level of interest in pain and the unique presence of nociceptive function within this group of thin sensory fibers, it is easy to conflate all A-delta and C fiber activity with pain exclusively, but this is an incorrect conclusion.[6]

Although some A-delta and C fibers are activated only by noxious or near-noxious heat or mechanical stimuli, most nociceptors respond during both types of stimulation, and some also respond to painful chemical stimulation; these are called "polymodal" nociceptors, responsive to more than one physically distinct stimulus or "modality" (e.g., thermal, mechanical, or chemical). An additional complication is that many, perhaps most, of these fibers show some low level of activity even before the stimulus intensity could be considered noxious. The results of these animal studies cloud our understanding of how the information provided by these nociceptors finally results in the human capacity to distinguish clearly different types of pain and to experience many different intensities and qualities of pain. What experience is associated with the activity of a polymodal nociceptor? Is there a "polymodal pain"? At what frequency of spike activity does a nociceptor produce pain? How many nociceptors does it take to produce pain?

PSYCHOPHYSICAL NEURONOGRAPHY

At about the time of publication of the discovery of putative nociceptors in the anesthetized cat, two researchers in Sweden published a brief report showing that they could record action potentials from the fibers of individual nerve cells in their own nerves. They inserted small recording probes (microelectrodes) through their skin and into their skin nerves to record the responses of single fibers to movements or to pressure applied to small skin areas.[7] The research potential of this technical advancement was immediately obvious; now it would be possible to correlate directly the activity of single sensory neurons in the human PNS with that person's sensory experience. We could investigate the mechanisms linking a measure of receptor activity with a qualitative and quantitative description of the resulting sensory experience. Put another way, we would be able, at least in theory, to determine the transfer function performed by the central nervous system (CNS) on the somatic sensory information presented by the PNS.

Near the time of the Issaquah meeting, reports of recording the action potentials of the smallest diameter sensory fibers from healthy, awake humans first appeared.[8] A few years later, experience and various technical improvements enabled human psychophysical and neurophysiological measurements to be combined so that a "nociceptor" could be characterized in terms of human experience. Figures 6.2 to 6.4 depict the results from

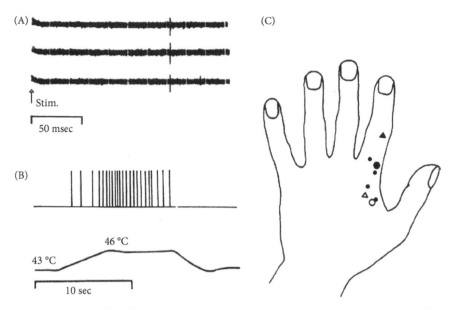

FIGURE 6.2. Electrophysiological recording of action potential firing from a single nociceptive fiber in the hand of a conscious human.

See text for explanation.

From Gybels J, Handwerker HO, and Van Hees J. A comparison between the discharges of human nociceptive nerve fibres and the subject's ratings of his sensations. *Journal of Physiology* 292: 193–206, 1979, Figure 1, with permission from John Wiley and Sons, Inc.

one of the first experiments to relate quantitatively the spike activity of single peripheral nerve fibers to measures of pain intensity.

Figure 6.2A shows three oscilloscope tracings of a voltage spike (action potential) recorded from a single fiber in the nerve innervating the left hand (C). In A, a painless electrical stimulus is applied to the skin of the knuckle of the index finger (designated by a *black triangle* in C) at the beginning (*left*) of each of the three oscilloscope traces. The recording from an electrode in the nerve at the wrist shows the spike response on the *right* of each trace at a fixed time (about 125 milliseconds) after each stimulus; this allows an estimation that the fiber's conduction velocity is in the range of C fibers. In B, a heat pulse rising from 43° C to 46° C is applied to the knuckle site, and the fiber action potentials trigger a train of electrical pulses shown above the heat pulse recording. In C, the symbols on the hand show the skin innervation sites from which electrical and heat stimuli evoked separate responses from eight individual C fibers; the *white* and *black triangles* and *larger circles* show the innervation sites of four fibers with stable recordings that allow a correlation of spike activity with the person's numerical rating of sensory experience.

Figure 6.3 is a line plot of the number of spikes generated by each of the eight single fibers at different temperatures of each heat stimulus. Each fiber generates more spikes as the stimulus temperature increases; some begin responding at 45° C and others at 46° C so that more fibers become active as the temperature increases. This result suggests that

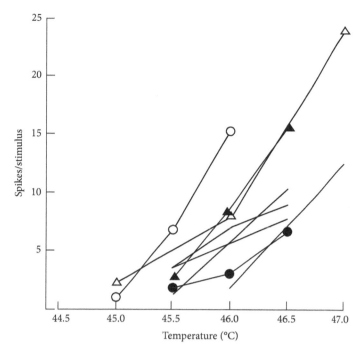

FIGURE 6.3. The action potential activity of each nociceptive fiber and the total number of active fibers increases with the intensity of heat applied to the skin areas (receptive fields) innervated by the fibers.

See text for explanation.

From Gybels J, Handwerker HO, and Van Hees J. A comparison between the discharges of human nociceptive nerve fibres and the subject's ratings of his sensations. *Journal of Physiology 292*: 193–206, 1979, Figure 2, with permission from John Wiley and Sons, Inc.

the "neural code" for heat pain intensity is the combined number of spikes generated by the fibers that are active at each temperature. In this small sample, none of the fibers is active at 44.1° C, the average temperature for "moderate" heat pain shown in the population histogram of Figure 6.1, but several are active at 45.6° C, the temperature for "moderate" pain determined in the other comparison psychophysical study cited earlier.

Figure 6.4 shows the spike activity of four fibers as a function of *perceived* heat stimulus intensity ("ratings"). (The activity of the fiber designated by *white triangles* is so high that it requires a separate vertical scale on the *right*.) There are six ratings of heat intensity, ranging from 1 (just noticeable heat) to 6 (very hot, painful). The transition from rating 3 to 4 indicates a change in sensory quality from "clearly warmer" (3) to "hot, slightly stinging" (4); between these ratings, there is an acceleration of total (cumulative) spike frequency, reflecting the abrupt increase in total spike activity between 45° C and 46° C seen in Figure 6.4.

Subsequent experiments (far too numerous to discuss or cite here) have confirmed these observations and extended them to include the small-diameter myelinated A-delta fibers, many of which also respond maximally to noxious heat and often have higher spiking frequencies than C fibers. Like C fibers, many A-delta fibers respond

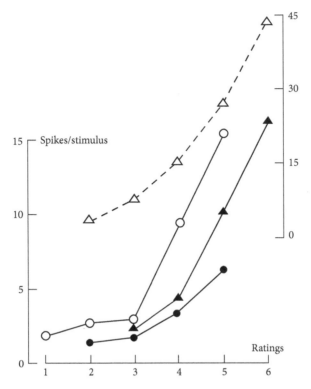

FIGURE 6.4. As the total number of action potentials increases, the perceived intensity of the applied heat stimulus increases. Some fibers become active before the heat becomes painful and others become active only during perceived pain.
See text for explanation.
From Gybels J, Handwerker HO, and Van Hees J. A comparison between the discharges of human nociceptive nerve fibres and the subject's ratings of his sensations. *Journal of Physiology* 292: 193–206, 1979, Figure 3, with permission from John Wiley and Sons, Inc.

to both heat and mechanical noxious stimuli; some also respond to noxious chemical stimuli. However, A-delta fibers appear to be more likely than C fibers to respond only to mechanical or thermal stimuli; some respond best to stimulation with a cold object or substance.[9]

As observed in recordings from animals, most nociceptors recorded from humans are "polymodal" to varying degrees. Sometimes, it may be difficult to detect clearly and quickly if a pain is mechanical, thermal, or chemical in origin, but the daily experience of most of us suggests that modality detection is not much of a problem. How this ambiguity in the PNS is resolved by the CNS is not clear. However, nociceptive C fibers responding only to mechanical or heat stimuli have been recorded from human skin nerves, so these fibers may contribute to the ability to identify the physical nature of the stimulus even during the activity of polymodal fibers.[10]

In thinking about pain mechanisms, it is important to realize that individual nociceptor activity is not always a faithful reflection of stimulus intensity. With prolonged stimulation, the spiking of some nociceptors may decline or even cease, although the applied stimulus intensity is unchanged. Alternatively, nociceptors may become sensitized by prolonged or repeated noxious stimulation so that their responses to noxious or even presumably innocuous stimuli become exaggerated. These response changes may or may not be associated with changes in perceived pain intensity. Changes in the activity of an individual fiber may be masked by continuing activity within a population of active nociceptive fibers; and integrative processes within the CNS can compensate for variations in the intensity of spike signals coming from sensory fibers.

Finally, the activity of a single nociceptive fiber may or may not result in pain or any sensation at all; this almost certainly depends, among many other variables, on its spike frequency. Moreover, it appears that a *population* of active nociceptive fibers is usually necessary for pain, at least as determined in the controlled laboratory setting exemplified by the experiments described previously. This conclusion is in accord with those based on recordings from whole intact nerves more than 80 years ago.[11] The critical size of this fiber population is unknown for the different types and locations of pain and for the many different circumstances in which noxious stimuli are encountered.

Overall, however, there is no doubt that, within the population of small-diameter myelinated and unmyelinated somatic sensory fibers (A-delta and C fibers), there are those that qualify as nociceptors as defined by the correlation of their activity with human reports of pain or "near pain" experiences. Most types of sudden-onset, relatively brief pain experienced in everyday life seem to be represented within this population.

We may therefore define a nociceptor as a peripheral sensory fiber with spike responses that correlate with a human's perception of pain—but we must limit the generality of this definition according to the circumstances under which the correlation is made. A laboratory is not a war zone, a clinic, an operating room, or a football field, where many other variables come into play; and most of us do not focus our daily lives on the detection of small changes in nociceptor activity. Pain is not simply X nociceptors spiking at Y frequency; there are many other determinants of pain.

INFLAMMATORY EXCITATION OF NOCICEPTORS AND NEUROGENIC INFLAMMATION

A critical feature of nociceptors is their response to and during inflammation, the biological response to tissue damage.[12] As the "flam" part of this word suggests, inflammation is a process that includes the generation of heat at the site of injury. The local heat is delivered by the rapid dilation of local blood vessels and the increased flow of warm blood to the site of injury. This response is triggered by damage to tissue-resident cells that release a rich and complex variety of organic molecules (e.g., proteins, peptides, lipids, polysaccharides) that, in turn, generate an equally complex cascade of other molecules that dilate blood vessels, increase the permeability of blood vessel membranes, and thus deliver even more blood-borne molecules and cells (e.g., white blood cells) to the site of injury. The local influx of blood, fluid, and cells produces local swelling as well as warmth. Medical and nursing students learn to recognize these events as three of the four cardinal clinical signs of inflammation: rubor (redness), calor (heat), and tumor (swelling). The fourth sign, of course, is dolor (pain), and this is where nociceptors come into the picture.

For obvious reasons, the inflammatory response of nociceptors is not easily studied in humans, so nearly all of the information about the response of nociceptors during inflammation comes from animal models. However, experimentally induced skin inflammation (mustard oil, capsaicin, carrageenan) in humans has shown that some C nociceptive fibers show inflammation-enhanced responses to heat or mechanical stimulation; indeed, some C fibers (called insensitive or silent nociceptors) begin to respond *only* during the induction of inflammation.[13]

As expected from the previous description of the inflammatory process, the initiation and maintenance of activity in an inflammation-responsive nociceptor depends on the chemical environment. And, alas, the chemical environment of inflammation is as complex as the inflammatory process itself. A recent review, for example, lists 18 different molecules (in addition to protons or hydrogen ions) as among the chemical constituents of the "inflammatory soup"[14] that excites nociceptors.[15] The inflammatory response also includes the participation of at least eight different tissue and blood cell types, each of which may add its own unique chemical cocktail into the mix of potential nociceptor activators. The activating components of the inflammatory soup then have varying degrees of access to at least five physiologically distinct membrane protein complexes, molecular sites that capture one or more of these activators. These membrane receptors directly or indirectly open ion channels in the nociceptor membrane, leading ultimately to the generation of action potentials that are propagated to the spinal cord and brainstem of the CNS.[16]

The complexity of the inflammatory excitation of nociceptors and spinal cord neurons is captured by the graphic depiction in Figure 6.5, which I have inserted here only to give the reader an intuitive grasp of the rich biology underlying the apparently simple act of injuring tissue. If you feel compelled to identify and understand the individual components of the highly interactive processes shown in this figure, you should consult the original article, which is a comprehensive review of molecular targets for the development of analgesic drugs. Otherwise, bear with me as I attempt to summarize the major concepts presented by this Figure.

The upper part of the figure shows the events that immediately follow tissue injury and the excitation of nociceptors. Several types of cells in the injured tissue (source, *top header, left*) release multiple inflammatory mediators (*top header, middle*) that bind to multiple receptors in the nociceptor membrane (peripheral terminal, *top header, right*), opening voltage-gated ion channels (Na x.x, Ca x.x) that lead to the generation of action potentials (*DRG* = dorsal root ganglion, the location of PNS nociceptor cell bodies). The drawing below the diagram depicts the anatomy of these processes.

The lower part of this figure summarizes events occurring in the dorsal gray matter of the spinal cord where spinal cord sensory neurons receive nociceptive input and send axons to the brainstem and thalamus. As depicted in the anatomical cartoon below the diagram, several neurotransmitters including neuropeptides are released into the spinal cord by the central endings of the nociceptive neuron shown on the *far left*; these in turn trigger the activity of three classes of cells within the spinal gray matter (spinal cells activated, *top header, middle*). The two types of non-neuronal cells (*resident* and *migrating*) release a variety of mediators of the inflammatory response *within* the spinal cord gray matter. (More about that later.) Spinal cord sensory neurons, which send axons to the

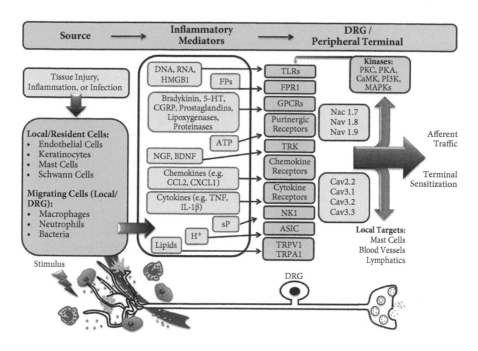

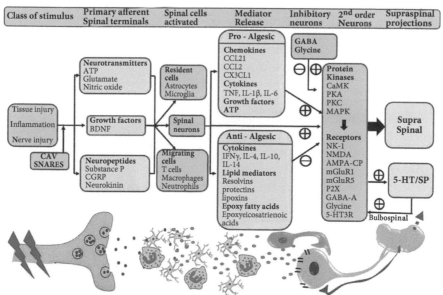

FIGURE 6.5. Diagrammatic representation of the inflammatory process in injured tissue (top) and of the accompanying neurochemical responses in the spinal cord gray matter. See original article for definition of labels in this figure.

See text for explanation.

From Yaksh TL, Woller SA, Ramachandran R, and Sorkin LS. The search for novel analgesics: Targets and mechanisms. *F1000Prime Reports* 7: 27, 2015. http://f1000.com/prime/reports/m/7/56.

brainstem and thalamus (supraspinal, *top header, far right*), are excited (e.g. glutamate) or inhibited (GABA, glycine) by neurotransmitters interacting with various inflammatory and protein mediators on multiple types of membrane receptors and ion channels (2nd order neurons, *top header, right*). This part of the figure also depicts some of the feedback onto spinal sensory neurons from nociceptively excited neurons in the brainstem (5-HT/ SP, brainstem drawing on *far right*).

If you're still with me after this elaboration, you should have a deeper appreciation of the complex and fascinating biology of tissue injury and the first steps toward pain. The chase for pain, however, continues to the brain. In any case, it should be apparent that the process of evolution has provided many paths and mechanisms for informing the CNS about the presence or threat of tissue damage.

In considering the implications of this complexity for the alleviation of pain, there are at least two closely related and somewhat conflicting viewpoints. One perspective, an optimistic one, is that there are many sites available for potential drug effects and thus opportunities for the development of new and perhaps more effective analgesic medicines. Indeed, this is a major point made by the authors of the article cited here and also by many others in the pharmacological and neuroscience communities. For example, a recent review of the inflammatory process in painful clinical disorders of peripheral nerves emphasizes the diagnostic and therapeutic promise of identifying, in patients, those components of the local inflammatory process that may be either analgesic or algesic (causing pain).[17]

A more cautionary assessment, also expressed by these and other authors, is that the multitude of participating cellular and molecular elements suggests that modifying the action of only one or a few of them will have a limited, perhaps clinically insignificant analgesic effect. Furthermore, the known or potential interactions among these agents and their known and potential effects on other biological systems make the field of analgesic development a minefield of unwelcome and potentially dangerous side effects. One example of this problem is the unfortunate discovery that an inhibitor of a pro-inflammatory enzyme (cyclooxygenase) also significantly increases the risk for stroke and heart attack.[18] The drug successfully attenuates inflammatory pain, but its effect on blood-clotting mechanisms has seriously restricted its widespread and prolonged use as an analgesic. Finally, all clinically effective anti-inflammatory analgesics in use today, such as aspirin and other nonsteroidal anti-inflammatory drugs (NSAIDs), have both PNS and CNS sites of action that reduce pain,[19] suggesting that focusing on only one site or mechanism of action is likely to be less successful than if more than one site of action is targeted for modification.

There is strong evidence that nociceptive fibers themselves contribute to inflammation through a process known as *neurogenic inflammation*, thus expanding the effects of inflammation and the inflammatory excitation of nociceptors. The peptide neurotransmitters that are released by nociceptive fibers into the dorsal spinal cord gray matter are also released into the tissue that the nociceptive fibers innervate, a kind of recoil effect.[20] These peptides can produce dilation and increased permeability of resident blood vessels, activate other inflammatory mediators, and sensitize the receptor endings of nearby nociceptive fibers. Neurogenic inflammation can amplify and prolong the inflammatory response to tissue damage; it also sensitizes the endings of nociceptors within or near the damaged tissue, making them responsive to stimuli that are usually painless (producing an experience called *allodynia*) or exaggerating their responses to painful stimuli (producing the experience of *hyperalgesia*). Allodynia and hyperalgesia lead to behavioral guarding of the injured site; in that sense, this *peripheral sensitization*[21] provides a protective function and facilitates healing. But if the tissue inflammation continues or if the nociceptor sensitization is prolonged, pain may become chronic and continue well beyond the time of healing. Chronic pain is also more likely to develop if, as discussed in Chapter 7, neurons within the CNS become sensitized also.

7

CENTRAL SENSITIZATION AND PAIN GENES

CENTRAL SENSITIZATION

A mild form of inflammation may also occur in the spinal cord and brain simply as the result of increased neuronal activity during the processing of nociceptive information. These central inflammatory mediators are shown in Figure 6.5. Like peripheral sensitization, this *central sensitization*, also called *neuroinflammation,* may be protective by facilitating the behavioral adaptation to injury or to increased metabolic demands. But in its more intense form, it may be maladaptive, leading to the release of pro-inflammatory substances from glial cells and other cellular components of the immune system.[1] In this latter condition, inflammation could be exaggerated and prolonged and could extend beyond the site of initiation to produce a pathological state of continued neuronal hyperexcitability in the central nervous system (CNS). The transition from acute to chronic pain could involve this neuroinflammatory process. Sensory input from the peripheral nervous system (PNS) that would normally be perceived as painless could then become painful. Low-frequency spikes emanating from injured tissue, from damaged nerve fibers, or even from non-nociceptive fibers might evoke pain.

What is the evidence that the activity of nociceptive fibers can produce CNS changes leading to painless stimulation becoming painful? Figure 7.1 depicts the result of an experiment that provides such evidence. Just as it is possible to record from single sensory fibers in a nerve, so will electrical microstimulation within a cutaneous nerve occasionally activate a single fiber and, in an attentive human, evoke a sensation that reflects the sensory function of that fiber. In Figure 7.1A, low-intensity electrical stimulation of a single, large-diameter fiber in a nerve at the ankle evokes a painless sensation of touch that is perceived as coming from a small area on the foot. (For example, try firmly and quickly rolling a finger over the nerve that runs between the bones of your elbow; you will probably feel a tactile sensation in your little finger; the "funny bone" effect.) In the experiment discussed here, capsaicin, the pungent substance in jalapeño peppers, is injected into the nearby skin, producing an area of mild inflammation, activity in small-diameter nociceptive fibers, and tactile tenderness. This area of tenderness to touch or pressure expands and encompasses the area of touch sensation evoked by electrical stimulation of the fiber. At that time (B), the identical low-intensity electrical stimulation of the single fiber produces, at that same location in the foot, a tactile sensation that is now accompanied, after a delay of one-half to one second, by a painful burning or stinging sensation in the same or nearby area. When the area of skin tenderness recedes (C), the single-fiber stimulation again evokes only a painless tactile sensation. Similar results were obtained in 11 of 14 other volunteers in this series of experiments. In interpreting

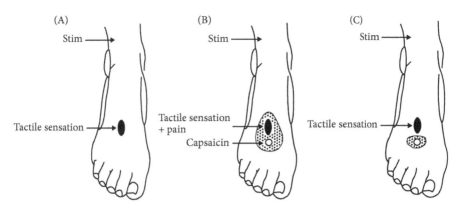

FIGURE 7.1. Capsaicin-induced inflammatory tenderness (painful touch, *dotted area* in B and C) changes the painless tactile sensation evoked in the foot (A, *black spot*) by electrical stimulation of a single fiber just above the ankle (*Stim*). When the area of induced tenderness expands into the area innervated by this fiber (B), the painless tactile sensation evoked by electrical stimulation of the same fiber is accompanied by a delayed (0.5 to 1 second) painful sensation of burning or stinging. The electrical stimulation again evokes only a painless tactile sensation when the area of tactile tenderness recedes (C). See text for further explanation and discussion.

From Torebjork HE, Lundberg LE, and LaMotte RH. Central changes in processing of mechanoreceptive input in capsaicin-induced secondary hyperalgesia in humans. *Journal of Physiology 448*: 765–780, 1992, with permission from John Wiley and Sons, Inc.

these results, it is important to realize that the change in sensation was caused by changes within the CNS because the unchanged low-intensity nerve stimulation was above the ankle, remote from the site of inflammation, and therefore continued to excite only the large-diameter nerve fibers that normally evoke a tactile sensation. The inflammatory activation of nociceptors had modified the central effect of these fibers.

Many other experiments in humans and animal models show that nociceptor activity generated by inflammation or other methods of prolonged nociceptor stimulation can change sensory processing in the CNS so that non-nociceptive sensory fibers can, at least temporarily, function like nociceptors. This effect can last for days or months in animal experiments and probably in humans with some chronic pain conditions. Whether this central sensitization is due to a mild form of neuroinflammation in the CNS is not known, but these results are at least consistent with that speculation.[2] It is reasonable to suggest that more serious and prolonged episodes of inflammation and nociceptor activation could produce longer lasting changes in CNS function, leading to the condition of *neuropathic pain* (discussed also in subsequent chapters) with chronic and intractable pain and exaggerated sensitivity to normally innocuous tactile or thermal stimuli even when the stimulus is applied outside the area of tissue damage (recall the cases of *causalgia* and *central pain* described earlier in the sample cases of pain experience).[3] It is possible that more commonly encountered forms of constant, chronic pain could be due in part to an exaggerated CNS sensitivity to normally unperceived ongoing background activity in small diameter A-delta and C fibers.[4]

Fortunately, central sensitization is usually treatable and not a frequent serious consequence of nociceptor activity. For example, the pain of chronic osteoarthritis is successfully relieved in the large majority of patients undergoing joint replacement surgery.[5] And in many other clinical conditions such as painful diabetic neuropathy or fibromyalgia, significant pain relief may be obtained with gabapentin or pregabalin, which, unlike anti-inflammatory or opioid drugs, are thought to reduce central sensitization specifically by suppressing calcium-mediated neurotransmission in CNS neurons receiving nociceptive input.[6] There is also good evidence that much of the pain attributed to sensitization of the CNS is sustained only when some degree of sensory fiber activity is present.[7] Thus, local anesthetics applied to painful areas can reduce or even eliminate the widespread, exaggerated sensitivity to noxious or innocuous stimulation.[8] Whether the PNS sensory input necessary to sustain central sensitization would be painful for a healthy person is unknown in most cases. However, in patients with causalgia or some similar cases of nerve injury pain, there is no doubt that normally innocuous somatic or even visual and auditory sensations produce or exaggerate the pain perceived as emanating from nearby uninjured areas. This extreme form of central sensitization may be caused by CNS neuroinflammation following a large, synchronous barrage from nerve fibers discharged by a missile impact or other sudden, direct nerve injury as in the case of causalgia described earlier. It is possible, but unproven, that some form of spontaneous, paroxysmal CNS neuroinflammatory-induced central sensitization is responsible for some common headache syndromes, especially migraine, which is frequently accompanied by heightened sensitivity to touch, light, and sound.

In other cases, however, it is likely that "top-down" influences from the brain or brainstem produce or sustain some degree of central sensitization.[9] For example, a series of experiments using a mouse model of pain behavior reveals a cingulate-to-insula circuit that appears to be necessary and sufficient for initiating and maintaining a state of central somatosensory sensitization that is independent of peripheral nociceptive input. These and functionally connected brain structures exert their modulating effect via a serotonin-mediated pathway to control sensory input at the level of the spinal cord.[10] (See also Chapter 8.)

Central sensitization is a form of *plasticity*, a term used to refer to the capacity of the CNS to adapt to environmental changes and to anatomical and physiological changes produced by normal neuronal activity or by injury to the PNS or CNS. A thorough discussion of neuronal plasticity involves learning, memory, and other topics well beyond the scope of this story. I will discuss this topic further in the context of brain imaging during acute and chronic pain.

GENETICS AND ION CHANNELS

There is no single "pain gene," one that alone codes for the entire neural mechanism mediating pain. The population distribution of pain thresholds (see Figure 5.2) is consistent with abundant evidence that many genes, the interactions among them, and the actions of molecular promoters and suppressors of genetic expression, act at many anatomical loci to determine whether a stimulus excites nociceptors and whether humans perceive that excitation as painful.[11] If, however, a "pain gene" is defined as a section of the deoxyribonucleic acid (DNA) molecule that participates in coding for proteins affecting pain-related behavior, then there are hundreds of pain genes. In fact, there is an interactive website (http://www.jbldesign.com/jmogil/enter.html), maintained by the pain research group at McGill University, that enables the user to search within the population of more than 400 pain genes identified thus far by gene suppression (or "knockout") experiments in mice. This website identifies the protein(s) associated with the gene and the type of behavioral test used to identify it as a pain-related gene. Another interactive website (http://www.PainNetworks.org) can be used to reveal the multiple interactions among pain genes and the proteins associated with them.[12] The link between a gene and a protein is maintained by a messenger form of ribonucleic acid (RNA) that transmits the code to a protein-manufacturing site within the cell; the integrity of this link is critical for assuring faithful transmission of the genetic instruction. The complexity of this genetic process means that, although there are many genetic targets for controlling pain, the clinical effect of each target is almost certain to be muted by the functional overlap and redundancy within the system. Pain seems to be hidden behind a fog of genes and the many proteins they help create.

An overriding problem with the strategy of guiding pain treatments by genetic functions is that proteins, the products of gene action, may number in the millions, but there are only an estimated 21,000 genes.[13] This numerical disparity guarantees that, on average, each gene participates in the construction and maintenance of multiple proteins. A mutation in a single gene may therefore have multiple effects, or it may be biologically silent. Gene actions can also influence one another so that a protein is likely to be affected by more than one gene. Nonetheless, the study of human genetic mutations that modify pain and painful conditions can suggest directions for research with therapeutic potential.

There is now evidence that nociceptive nerve fibers have unique ion channels that could serve as biochemical markers of nociceptive function and possibly as future targets for therapeutic intervention. Studies of rare cases of *congenital insensitivity (or indifference) to pain* and of several *inherited painful conditions* have led to the discovery of genes that encode for proteins making up specific ion channels (especially for sodium) found primarily and perhaps only in the membranes of nociceptive nerve fibers. Mutations in these genes, even in a single gene, can lead to structural changes in the proteins comprising the channel, producing either a gain of channel function with increased pain or a loss of channel function with a loss or attenuation of pain. For example, one type of mutation in a single gene leads to a congenital insensitivity only to pain, while different mutations *in the same gene* produce two different familial inherited disorders with spontaneous paroxysms of intense pain. This particular gene encodes for the production of a protein in a biochemically and structurally unique sodium channel that directly affects neuronal excitability.[14] Recent studies in rodents have shown that antibodies directed against a protein within this particular channel can reduce pain and itching behaviors without affecting tests of motor function.[15] Whether this type of antibody treatment could work in humans remains to be determined and will surely require extensive and prolonged studies. One problem with this strategy is that there are additional sodium channels that have been identified as being primarily or uniquely present in the membranes of nociceptive fibers.[16] Targeting one particular channel may not be sufficient to achieve a clinically significant effect. Furthermore, at least one of these channels is found in the membranes of the ganglia of neurons in the sympathetic part of the autonomic nervous system in mice (see autonomic nervous system in the Appendix), raising the possibility that changing its function could have widespread side effects in humans.

Another problem is that there are likely to be several different genetic mutations that lead to different clinical conditions with abnormally high or even unobtainable pain thresholds. The previous ambiguous reference to congenital *insensitivity or indifference* to pain reflects the history of case reports in the clinical literature. Currently, *insensitivity* has become associated with a genetically determined and microscopically identifiable loss of A-delta and C fibers in sensory nerves or the spinal cord, often associated with impairments of cognition or autonomic functions like sweating. These associated abnormalities are absent in most of the reported cases that have been labeled *indifference* to pain because, in the "indifference" cases, all other neurological functions, including the ability to discriminate among heat, cold, and mechanical stimuli, are intact. Therefore, it is possible that at least some previously reported cases of indifference actually have a genetically determined ion channel abnormality or "channelopathy" as discussed earlier[17]; others may have anatomical or functional abnormalities, perhaps in the CNS, that have yet to be discovered.

But a primary concern, from both clinical and economic perspectives, is the development of chronic pain and its treatment. It is possible that, in the near future, genetic information will play an important role in preventing chronic pain. There is some evidence that an individual's genetic profile can be a factor in determining the vulnerability for developing some types of chronic pain.[18] Although the presumably responsible genes are hardwired into the genetic profile and cannot be altered easily, some of them could be detected by appropriate genetic testing so that medical interventions with an increased risk for chronic pain could be modified or avoided. In addition, the expression of a gene's action (the phenotype) can be modified by various environmental stresses, some of which can modify genetic material (DNA) itself in the prenatal, postnatal, and early stages of development. Some of these *epigenetic* influences may predispose an individual to chronic pain, so particular care could be taken to avoid these stressors if there is an at-risk genetic profile. Finally, it is all but certain that much of the vulnerability for chronic pain occurs because of the genetically programmed development of specific CNS circuits that increase or decrease the neuronal signals leading to pain. Detecting abnormal activity within and among these *pain-modulating* circuits could also help prevent the development of chronic pain and even facilitate its treatment. All the aforementioned gene-related interventions are now largely if not entirely hypothetical. However, given the rapid pace and increasing availability of genetic analysis and brain imaging technologies, the implementation of these procedures may not be very far away.[19]

8

CENTRAL NERVOUS SYSTEM MODULATION
OF PAIN
NEUROPHYSIOLOGICAL
AND CLINICAL EVIDENCE

As previously noted, the concept that brain activity and various "psychological" states affect pain perception was widely accepted well before the time of the Issaquah meeting. The examples given at the beginning of this story are clear indications that "states of mind" can have profound attenuating or amplifying effects on pain. The report of Henry K. Beecher, a pioneering anesthesiologist at Harvard, is often cited in the pain research literature as another example of pain modulation by environmental circumstances prevailing at the time of serious injury. During his service in World War II, Beecher noted that a majority (76 of 150; 51%) of severely wounded soldiers, although fully alert and cooperative, rated their pain as slight or absent, and only 32% requested analgesic treatment after being removed from the battlefield to the field hospital. By contrast, 113 (75%) of an identical number of peace-zone community civilians with similar or even less severe traumatic or surgical wounds rated their pain as moderate or severe, and most (83%) requested analgesic medication. Beecher attributed these results to differences in the "reaction component" of pain. The soldiers, he speculated, likely considered their wounds as events that removed them from battle, thus sparing them from more serious injury or death. He thought that the civilians were more likely to view their wounds as significant threats to their health and livelihood. For Beecher, these different cognitive processes led to contrasting interpretations of the significance of similar wounds and somehow reduced pain for the soldiers—but not for the civilians, who might even have had an *increased* pain sensitivity. In a subsequent scholarly review, Beecher discussed and summarized the multiple environmental determinants of perceived pain intensity, emphasizing the importance of emotional and cognitive factors surrounding a painful illness or injury and their effects on the response to treatment.[1] It is notable, however, that he considered these factors to be modifying the "reaction component" *to* pain rather than acting directly on the neural mechanisms that produce the experience of pain.

SOME ANALGESIA CIRCUITS

The concept of direct central nervous system (CNS) control over pain was developing more secure physiological and anatomical support at the time of the Issaquah meeting, but it was still largely an observed behavioral phenomenon with limited neurophysiological and neuroanatomical detail about mechanisms. Earlier neurophysiological studies had shown that electrical stimulation in the brain or brainstem and changes in the level of alertness could change the tactile and nociceptive responses of sensory neurons in the spinal cord and thalamus.[2] Later, recordings from individual neurons in the brainstem dorsal gray matter of awake, trained monkeys revealed that attention, predictability, and reward anticipation modified the responses of CNS neurons that receive input directly from nociceptive fibers in the peripheral nervous system (PNS). This was the first and most direct evidence that high-level cerebral processes modified nociceptive information at the earliest stage of transmission in the CNS.[3] Still, the CNS circuitry mediating these changes was poorly understood, and the supporting evidence relied heavily on studies of anesthetized animals and the interpretation of animal behavior. Critical information that could link human experience to the neurophysiology of pain and analgesia was lacking.

The Periaqueductal Gray Connection

The seminal discovery that electrical stimulation within the brains of animals could reduce or eliminate behavioral responses to noxious stimuli (*nocifensive responses*) without obviously disturbing other behaviors or general alertness led to a series of studies confirming and extending these findings and focusing attention on the central gray matter of the rostral brainstem (periaqueductal gray, or PAG) and its connections

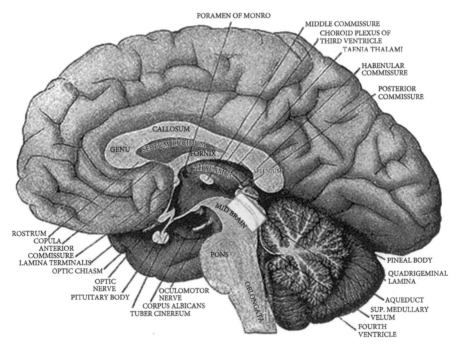

FIGURE 8.1. The location of the periaqueductal gray matter is indicated by the *yellow rectangle* in the upper part of the brainstem.
(Figure extracted and modified from Figure A.4 in the Appendix.)

(Figure 8.1).[4] The PAG comprises brainstem neurons (the "gray matter") and supporting glial cells surrounding a midline tubular conduit (the aqueduct) that connects the fluid-filled large ventricles of the cerebral hemispheres with the fluid surrounding the brainstem and spinal cord (the cerebrospinal fluid, or CSF). In humans, this structure, located deep within the CNS, is approximately 14 millimeters (one-half inch) long and 5 millimeters (three-sixteenths inch) wide. Anatomically distinct columns of nerve cells extend throughout the long axis of the PAG, sending and receiving axons to and from the spinal cord, brainstem, and hypothalamus. Parts of the PAG send axons to the central part of the thalamus, which has connections with limbic system structures in the brain; these, in turn, send axons back to the PAG, forming a feedback loop that typifies most connections within the CNS. Because of these anatomical connections, PAG neurons as a group can affect and modify many functions, including pain, emotional responses (e.g., anxiety and fear), sexual behavior, and unconscious (autonomic) body functions such as micturition, heart rate, and blood pressure.[5] Because many of the anti-nocifensive stimulation sites are located within the lower (ventral) part of the PAG, and because an earlier study had shown that destructive lesions within the PAG attenuated nocifensive behavior in cats,[6] this small structure became the focus of intensive investigation for more than two decades. The studies confirmed earlier findings that electrical stimulation within the lower (ventral) part of the PAG produced an apparently selective anti-nocifensive effect in awake rats because the putatively analgesic area was often localized to only part of the body. Subsequent research revealed opioid receptors in the PAG and showed that the direct microinjection of opioid compounds produced an anti-nociception that was blocked by the injection of specific opioid receptor antagonists into the PAG. Destruction of parts of the PAG reduced or eliminated the anti-nocifensive effect of morphine-like drugs. Neuronal recording and anatomical studies showed further that the anti-nocifensive effects of PAG activity depended on its connections to neurons in the center of the lower brainstem (the medial medulla) just above (rostral to) the spinal cord. Some neurons in this medial medullary area developed increased activity just before a lightly anesthetized rat reflexively withdrew its tail from noxious heat (the tail-flick reflex); these neurons were called "on cells." The counterpart of the "on cell" was, of course, the "off cell," which was continuously (tonically) active until about one-half second before the tail flick. As expected, morphine-like opioid drugs turned on cells off and off cells on. Neuronal recording studies showed that activation of this PAG-medullary circuit inhibited spinothalamic tract neurons in the dorsal gray matter of the spinal cord. Finally, as noted previously, this PAG-medullary circuit receives neuronal input from several brain areas, including components of the limbic system such as the hypothalamus and the cingulate cortex in the frontal lobe. Subsequent studies showed that other circuits connect the brain and brainstem and use other neurotransmitters (e.g., dopamine, serotonin, and norepinephrine) to reduce the activity of nociceptive spinothalamic tract neurons. Here, then, were circuits that could not only explain at least part of the mechanisms mediating the action of the most effective analgesic drugs, including the opioid narcotics, but also how the brain, by independently and naturally activating these built-in (endogenous) circuits and their neurochemical mediators, could profoundly modulate pain.[7]

Diffuse Noxious Inhibitory Control

There is strong evidence from studies in animal models and in humans that noxious stimulation in one part of the body reduces nocifensive responses (and pain in humans) to noxious stimulation elsewhere, a phenomenon called *diffuse noxious inhibitory control*, or DNIC. DNIC is mediated by a loop consisting of nociceptive responses that ascend in the ventrolateral spinal cord (with the crossed spinothalamic tract) and activate brainstem reticular formation neurons (separate from the PAG) that suppress nociceptive responses of sensory neurons on both sides of the spinal cord. For example, in a patient with a traumatic (knife wound) hemisection of the left thoracic spinal cord, spinal nociceptive reflexes in the arms (above the lesion) were suppressed by noxious conditioning stimulation of the two other limbs but *not* of the right foot. (This patient also had increased pain [hyperalgesia] and reflexes in the left leg below the cord lesion, consistent with a loss of descending inhibition and Brown-Sequard's earlier observation.[8]) Why the DNIC mechanism should have survived evolutionary challenges is a matter of speculation, but it may provide a kind of sensory filtering function that enhances the signal generated by activity in nociceptive nerve fibers[9]; also, it may contribute to the perceived pain-alleviating effects of counter-irritation folk remedies such as cupping, acupuncture, and mustard plaster.

However, caveats must be applied to the previous story of putative analgesia circuits.[10] First, it is important to note that most of the behavioral tests for pain are performed in animal models using spinal reflexes or other rapid withdrawal responses to noxious stimuli applied while the animal is lightly anesthetized. These behaviors can be modified by inhibitory and excitatory synapses acting on spinal neurons (motor neurons) that directly excite muscles without affecting sensation or input from sensory fibers of the PNS. Therefore, although it is known that these brainstem neurons, including "on" and "off" cells, send their axons to both sensory and motor neurons in the spinal cord gray matter, the reduced nocifensive behaviors seen in these animal studies could be due to an effect on motor as well as sensory function. Second, as suggested by the presence of "on" cells, the brainstem sites that produce anti-nociception also include neurons that *facilitate* nocifensive behaviors, a kind of anti-analgesia or possible pain facilitation. As noted in Chapter 7), some brain structures that are activated during pain or analgesia form circuits that can initiate and sustain somatosensory central sensitization and pain via brainstem pathways that employ serotonin as a neurotransmitter.[11] Again, although there is some uncertainty about the degree to which these changes in nocifensive behaviors are mediated by actions on motor or sensory spinal neurons, the likelihood is that both effects are active under various circumstances and conditions during the course of normal living. Third, there is evidence that the PAG-rostral medullary circuit is not simply an analgesia system; rather, neurons in these structures, including "on" and "off" cells, appear to participate in several homeostatic functions such as thermoregulation, visceral motor control (urination, defecation), and levels of sleep and wakefulness. The control over sensory input exhibited by these neurons is not limited to nociception but includes tactile and visceral inputs as well. Their widely distributed effects may reflect a broad regulatory function that includes adjusting sensory input according to tissue condition and behavioral state. Finally, it is important to note that the PAG and the brainstem reticular neurons mediating DNIC receive input directly from the spinothalamic tract,[12] suggesting that, under normal circumstances, these structures participate in *feedback mechanisms* (discussed further later) that regulate sensory and motor responses to nociceptive input at the spinal cord level. These spinal reflexes can contribute to the initiation and execution of voluntary protective behaviors. Thus, artificial interference with these control systems (by anatomical, pharmacological, or electrical manipulation) could impair not only sensory functions but also the regulation of reflex excitability and voluntary responses to noxious stimuli.

STIMULATING ANALGESIA CIRCUITS IN HUMANS

As one might expect, shortly after the discovery of PAG-induced anti-nociception, neurosurgeons implanted stimulating electrodes aimed for the PAG and other structures (deep brain stimulation, or DBS) in an attempt to provide pain relief for patients with chronic, intractable pain of various causes.[13] Aside from the risks for infection and local brain trauma, applying electrical current within the PAG or the more rostral gray matter has mixed and often undesirable effects. Some patients report a significant degree of relief from the pain of their clinical condition, but others complain of very unpleasant side effects, such as feelings of fear, dread, or nausea often accompanied by changes in blood pressure; these results are not surprising given the biologically nonselective, artificial character of electrical stimulation and the extensive connections of the PAG with the hypothalamus and other limbic system structures. Locating the stimulating electrodes to other sites, such as the medial or lateral thalamus or the cingulate cortex, sometimes has therapeutic and side effects that are similar but seem to depend on the various characteristics and causes of the patient's pain. Overall, the percentage of patients with various causes of pain who receive some degree of benefit from stimulating various structures, including the PAG and the nearby periventricular gray matter (PVG), is typically in the range of 60% or less—even in a small, carefully selected group of patients. Because of its risks, side effects, and variable efficacy, DBS is currently offered to a very small percentage of patients with severe chronic pain that has proved resistant to other forms of medical and surgical intervention.

The promise of selectively and artificially activating pain inhibitory circuits by DBS thus faces constraints imposed by the interaction of CNS circuits that create pain, pain modulation, and pain-related experiences. A somewhat less invasive approach is electrical or pulsed magnetic stimulation applied to the fibrous covering of the brain (the dura) or to the scalp overlying the motor area of the cerebral cortex.[14] The physiological rationale for attempting to stimulate this cortical area for pain relief was suggested by the results of animal neurophysiological experiments. Although the evidence suggests that the motor cortical neurons are very weakly stimulated at the intensities typically used, the term "motor cortex stimulation" (MCS) is used to refer to this treatment. As applied to patients, primarily those with pain following CNS damage from stroke (central poststroke pain, or CPSP), MCS provides a variable and generally modest, usually temporary, attenuation of pain in about half of the patients with CPSP and other forms of pain caused by damage to the spinal cord or peripheral nerves. The neurophysiological basis for pain attenuation by MCS is unclear, but recent human brain imaging studies (discussed later) indicate that it affects the activity of other cortical and subcortical structures that are *excited* by noxious stimuli (e.g., anterior cingulate and orbitofrontal cortex, thalamus, and the PAG). This apparent paradox suggests that brain structures that are excited during pain also participate in a *feedback mechanism* that can attenuate pain. Again, as in the neurophysiology of DNIC and of pain facilitation ("on" vs. "off" cells), we recognize the presence of feedback control mechanisms[15] as part of the CNS mechanism for the modulation of pain and nocifensive behavior.

STIMULATING PAIN GENERATION CIRCUITS IN HUMANS

If pain can be reduced or increased by stimulation within the brain, can pain be produced directly, not simply increased, by stimulation within the brain? Yes,[16] but the sites from which pain has been evoked are quite limited due, in part, to the organization of the brain but also to the infrequent occasions when it is medically acceptable to use electrical stimulation in the course of identifying brain or other CNS sites for neurosurgical therapy. Keep in mind the possibility that electrical stimulation can excite the pathways leading to and from, as well as within, the site of stimulation. As would be expected, it is possible to evoke pain by electrical stimulation in the spinothalamic tract in the spinal cord and at its termination in the lateral (outer) and medial (inner) parts of the thalamus. Rare cases of patients with pain as a component of an epileptic seizure have been found to have an excitable focus in the insular cortex, leading eventually to the demonstration that electrical stimulation within the posterior dorsal (upper) part of this cortex and the adjacent "secondary" somatosensory cortex (S2) can evoke pain (at about 11% of more than 500 stimuli at these sites among 164 patients undergoing surgery for epilepsy; see Figure 8.2). Electrical stimuli applied within the primary somatosensory cortex of the postcentral gyrus has not evoked pain, but thus far the stimulation sites have not included the portion of this cortex containing the NS-type neurons mentioned previously.[17] The aforementioned pain-evoking sites are within two or three synaptic relays of the normal input from PNS nociceptors, so they may represent an early stage in the neurophysiological elaboration of pain. Like the PNS nociceptors, their excitation naturally engages many additional CNS neurons in multiple sites to establish the full pain experience. Accordingly, there are likely to be other CNS locations from which pain or unpleasant somatic (or visceral) sensations can be evoked, but these have yet to be identified. Finally, recalling the ubiquitous feedback control organization within the CNS, it must be noted that injury or disease affecting these pain-evoking sites is often associated with the onset of continuous central pain as experienced by Salvatore and J.J. in the introductory sample of pain experiences (see Chapter 1).[18] Damage of the nociceptive system often has at least two concurrent consequences: hypalgesia and chronic pain.

So, if pain can be modified by CNS activity and produced by stimulation within the CNS, what structures are affected by these manipulations? The evidence discussed thus far shows that pain does not have a single location; rather, it emerges from the activity of several structures in the brain. As we have seen, the information from PNS nociceptors is distributed among many structures—and destroying or injuring one CNS structure or pathway does not eliminate pain permanently. The fact that pain can be evoked by applying electrical stimulation within the insula, for example (see Figure 8.2), means

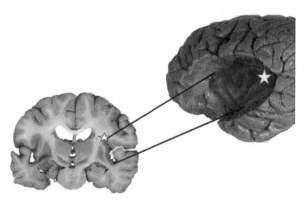

FIGURE 8.2. The insular (island) cortex, shown here in *red*, is an infolding of the cerebral cortex that covers the outside of the brain. A cross-section of the brain through the insula is shown at the lower left and a dissected left hemisphere is at the upper right, showing the insula with its five folds (gyri) exposed after removal of the overlying cortex. The S2 cortex is perpendicular and adjacent to the upper pole of the insula as shown in the cross-section. Pain was evoked by electrical stimulation within S2 and the insular area indicated by the *yellow stars* (Mazzola L, Isnard J, Peyron R, and Mauguiere F. Stimulation of the human cortex and the experience of pain: Wilder Penfield's observations revisited. *Brain 135*: 631–640, 2012). The insula, because of its unique evolutionary history and immediate connections with components of the somatosensory, limbic, and autonomic nervous systems, is considered by some to be a critical component of the mechanisms generating self-awareness, emotion, and feeling states generally, including the hedonic component of pain (Craig AD. How do you feel—now? The anterior insula and human awareness. *Nature Reviews Neuroscience 10*: 59–70, 2009; Craig AD. The sentient self. *Brain Structure and Function 214*: 563–577, 2010; Damasio AR, Grabowski TJ, Bechara A, Damasio H, Ponto LL, Parvizi J, and Hichwa RD. Subcortical and cortical brain activity during the feeling of self-generated emotions. *Nature Neuroscience 3*: 1049–1056, 2000).
Figure modified and obtained online in compliance with open access policies of StudyBlue.com and slideshare.net.

that this structure is part of a brain circuit that can generate pain, but it does *not* mean that the insula alone produces pain—or is even necessary (to be discussed later). Still, the identification of structures and pathways that make up part of a pain-generating circuit can be critically important for making clinical decisions and in guiding research. After the Issaquah meeting, some technical advances enabled studies that provide additional information about the anatomy and physiology of pain-related circuits.

ELECTROPHYSIOLOGICAL IDENTIFICATION OF PAIN-RELATED CIRCUITS

The invention and production of the *infrared* laser led to using this device to stimulate heat-sensitive nociceptors selectively, rapidly, and synchronously with very brief (about 1 millisecond) heat pulses focused on a small spot of skin (e.g., 5 mm diameter). The resulting synchronous barrage of action potentials in A-delta and C fibers gives a pinprick sensation (from the myelinated A-delta fibers) followed by a lower intensity and longer duration warmth or burning sensation (from the unmyelinated C fibers). Mechanically sensitive fibers are not stimulated by this type of laser, so this method produces a pure heat sensation and a thermo-selective excitation of CNS structures and pathways, such as the spinothalamic tract. The temporal coherence of the barrage of nociceptive fiber action potentials generates synchronous synaptic activity in the CNS structures first receiving it. The electrical response of these CNS structures can be measured as an "evoked potential," a sudden change of voltage recorded from electrodes on the human scalp. This laser-evoked potential (LEP) appears following heat stimulation at painful pinprick intensities and is shown in Figure 8.3. Note that the LEP responses (from both A-delta and C fiber stimulation) are widely distributed over the head, consistent with the distribution of nociceptive neuronal responses among several structures on both sides of the brain (i.e., bilaterally). The application of special neurophysiological analysis programs shows that the distribution of the LEP is best explained by neuronal responses occurring bilaterally in the areas of the S2 and insula cortices, with some contribution from the cingulate cortex near the midline of the brain. This type of

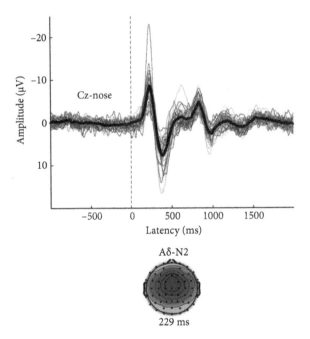

FIGURE 8.3. *Top:* The averaged laser-evoked potentials (LEPs) recorded from the center of the scalp from 34 normal individuals following the stimulation (at latency time of 0 milliseconds) of A-delta and C fibers in a small skin area of one hand. The *heavy black line* is the group average; the *many colored lines* are individual averages. The LEP amplitude (μV, ± microvolts) is the voltage difference between the center of the head (*Cz*) and the nose. The early large-amplitude wave is due to - delta fiber stimulation; the later and next largest wave is due to C fiber stimulation. *Below:* The spatial distribution of the early negative phase of the A-delta LEP (Aδ-N2) at its peak latency (229 milliseconds) is shown in amplitude-dependent *blue shading* over the top of a head diagram (nose up). The distribution of the C LEP is similar. The laser stimulus was perceived as a painful pinprick sensation that increased in intensity as the amplitude of the A-delta LEP increased.

Adapted from Hu L, Cai MM, Xiao P, Luo F, and Iannetti GD. Human brain responses to concomitant stimulation of Adelta and C nociceptors. *Journal of Neuroscience 34:* 11439–11451, 2014 with permission of the Society for Neuroscience.

analysis, however, is largely limited to the cerebral cortex, depends heavily on the location and spatial orientation of cortical neurons, and therefore underestimates the extent of nociceptor-related responses. A method with a high spatial resolution for localizing laser-evoked responses is magnetoencephalography (MEG), which records the magnetic fields generated by current flow around responding neurons. MEG recordings also show that the S1, S2, insular, and cingulate cortices contribute to the generation of the LEP, but they are likewise strongly affected and limited by the spatial orientation of active cortical neurons. Nonetheless, despite its limitations in spatial localization, studies of the LEP reveal some of the important variables affecting pain perception and can be used as an indicator of activity in pain-generating neurons. For example, LEP amplitude varies with the intensity of heat nociceptor activity and with changes in the perceived intensity of pain.

The amplitudes of both the A-delta and C components of the LEP are reduced by innocuous brushing at the site of laser stimulation, consistent with the common experience of pain relief by rubbing an injured site. And, like pain, LEP amplitude is strongly affected by the degree of alertness and by cognitive factors such as attention, expectation, stimulus salience, and the placebo effect (discussed in Chapter 10).[19]

Electromagnetic responses such as the LEP are useful biological indicators (biomarkers) of neuronal responses to stimuli that excite nociceptors specifically. As noted here, their amplitude varies with stimulus intensity and is sensitive to cognitive variables that affect perceived pain intensity. Contemporary analytical methods can provide some information about the location of the neurons that generate these responses, but the spatial resolution and specificity of these methods is quite limited.

A significant limitation of these evoked response approaches is that they sample neuronal responses over a very short span of time, typically less than a second. Clinically significant pain lasts much longer, of course, and is likely to have a quantitative and qualitative dynamic reflecting the recruitment of different structures over time. This temporal dynamic limitation can be at least partially overcome by the application of methods that analyze the rhythmic activity of groups of neurons over several seconds, minutes, or even longer. Group rhythmic activity (called *gamma oscillations*) can be recorded from the surface of the head as changes in voltage (the electroencephalogram, or EEG) or as changes in the magnetic field (MEG) generated by the flow of synaptically generated currents across neuronal membranes (dendrites and cell bodies). The existence of these rhythms means that large groups of neurons in the cerebral cortex are in synchronous activity, communicating with one another through connections that can vary widely in length, strength, and rhythmic frequency. By monitoring and measuring changes in the amplitude, frequency, and synchrony of these group rhythms, we can obtain estimates of connectivity, and of changes in connectivity, among whole neuronal populations under a variety of conditions including pain[20] (discussed further in Chapter 11). Measuring connectivity, however, is of very limited value without information about when and where these connections are being made. The development of anatomical and functional CNS imaging, discussed in Chapters 9 and 10, provides an opportunity to investigate these dynamics among anatomically identifiable CNS circuits.

WHEN CONTROL BREAKS DOWN

Pain normally begins with, and is sustained by, the excitation of nociceptors in body tissues. In fact, the connection between pain and the excitation of nociceptors and their impulse-conducting A-delta and C nerve fibers is typically so robust that these fibers are commonly called "pain fibers." But the evidence presented earlier leaves no doubt that the brainstem and brain contain anatomically and physiologically identifiable inhibitory and excitatory circuitry that has a dominating influence on pain, not simply on the "re-action to pain" but on the neuronal mechanisms leading to the experience of pain itself. Nonetheless, there are limits to these CNS controls. For many common pain experiences, the intensity and duration of nociceptive input may be too great; CNS controls simply cannot stop the pain of drilling into a tooth or of burning a finger. The endogenous pain control mechanisms may be overwhelmed by excessive nociceptive input and the activation of affective mechanisms.

Furthermore, when the CNS or PNS is injured or genetically altered, normal pain control mechanisms may be impaired so that the relation between tissue damage and nociceptive activity pain breaks down. Individuals with certain genetic abnormalities that prevent the excitation of nociceptive fibers do not feel the pain of tissue damage. At the other extreme, patients with different mutations in the same gene experience paroxysms of severe pain but without tissue damage. Much more common is the pain that sometimes follows damage to either the CNS or PNS; it is unlike the familiar and commonplace pain of tissue injury, however painful that may be; rather, it is an abnormal, pathological pain caused by the impairment of endogenous nociceptive control systems---it is *neuropathic pain*.[21] Patients with severe, sudden nerve injury or prolonged nociceptive input may, because of central sensitization, experience normally painless sensory activity as excruciating. Following central sensitization, abnormal spontaneous activity that is often generated in damaged nerves may be perceived as painful. Nerve damage can also change the normal mixture of active myelinated and unmyelinated sensory fibers, thus altering the balance of their excitatory and inhibitory effects within the CNS. Damage to nociceptive mechanisms within either the CNS or PNS can interrupt normal nociceptive feedback control mechanisms, leading to the seemingly paradoxical condition, seen in many of the central pain syndromes (see Chapter 1), in which pain is perceived continuously in a body area that is hypalgesic to stimuli that are normally painful. Neuropathic pain, when severe, is perhaps the most challenging painful condition facing patients, nurses, and physicians. Because an important component of neuropathic pain is due to changes in the CNS, we must learn more about how the CNS processes the nociceptive information it receives both normally and under pathological conditions. In seeking this medical goal, we may also gain important insights into the CNS mechanisms underlying other sensory, motor, mnemonic, and cognitive functions—the neuroscientific goal. And because pain occurs only in the conscious brain, we may even touch on the persistent philosophical problem of how the brain produces consciousness. But to make progress toward these goals, we need to *locate and measure* neuronal activity as impulses from nociceptors travel within the CNS. For this, we need to see the brain.

9

CENTRAL NERVOUS SYSTEM GENERATION
AND MODULATION OF PAIN
EARLY EVIDENCE FROM ANATOMICAL BRAIN
IMAGING AND THE DEVELOPMENT
OF FUNCTIONAL BRAIN IMAGING

ANATOMICAL IMAGING: COMPUTED TOMOGRAPHY
AND MAGNETIC RESONANCE IMAGING

The impact of imaging the brain and other parts of the central nervous system (CNS) in living humans has been broad and deep. Formerly hidden from view, and consequently shrouded in a kind of mystery, the living, human CNS, and the brain especially, are now revealed by images that are commonplace, seen in popular magazines, newspapers, and on television throughout the world. Today, brain function is sometimes the subject of discussion on radio and television talk shows. Gradually, the idea that the function of this organ determines what all humans and other animals feel and how they behave is increasingly common. How all this will affect our relationships with one another remains to be seen, but over time, it has the potential to be helpful.

Before the 1980s, the only way we could see any part of the brain of a living person or animal was during neurosurgical operations that opened the skull. Otherwise, the living brain was invisible. The structure of the brain could be studied only when it was extracted from the skull of the deceased. The function of structures composing the brain, such as parts of the cerebral cortex, thalamus, basal ganglia, brainstem, and spinal cord, could only be inferred from the deficits detected by the examination or simply by obser-vation of individuals (humans and other animals) who had sustained damage within the structures of interest. And, to a significant degree, this strategy worked; it allowed the clinician, simply by performing a clinical examination on a patient, to make a reasonable estimate of the location of the lesion. The accuracy of this estimation varied widely and depended heavily on the location and size of the lesion and the details and focus of the examination. The validation of this estimation depended on the availability of the CNS at autopsy, however, and this was highly variable and became increasingly rare during the late 20th century. But the method of localizing disease by clinical examination (i.e., *clinical localization*) was the only one available, and it worked well enough to be established as standard medical practice for the clinical investigation of disorders of the nervous system.

When clinical localization worked (i.e., it predicted the autopsy findings), it reinforced the conceptual model of functional localization as the basis for clinical practice, as a foundation for basic research, and as a focal point for various philosophical discussions about the mind. When clinical localization did not work, the failure was either ignored, chalked up to a limitation of the examination (or examiner), or, less often, recognized as an inconvenient limitation of the conceptual model. The idea that serious and important neurological functions (like pain) could not be localized consistently by examination, even with ancillary tests such as electroencephalography, met with resistance or silent denial. As noted here in previous sections, experiments and clinical observations during the late 19th century and early 20th century (e.g., Brown-Sequard, Broca, and their critics) suggested some limitations of the functional localization model of the time, but the model worked often and well enough to sustain it.

The invisibility of the living brain forced clinicians to use various invasive procedures to detect, with x-ray images, distortions of the CNS by visualizing the spaces and blood vessels surrounding the anatomical areas of interest. These procedures involved the injection of radiographic contrast liquid into blood vessels or air into spaces around the brain or spinal cord; they were uncomfortable, even painful, and carried risks of serious complications. Because of these clinical considerations, computerized tomography[1] (CT) was developed, based on a working physical model constructed in the early 1960s and fully implemented in the late 1970s, resulting in the Nobel Prize for Physiology or Medicine.[2]

With the development of the CT scanner, the living brain became visible. Clinicians and researchers could then begin identifying, within living individuals, brain locations associated with brain functions, including pain. It soon became clear that, although many lesions in various locations had no effect on pain, brain lesions that affected pain also impaired other neurological functions.[3] CT scanning revealed that small lesions in the thalamus produced losses of tactile, vibratory, and kinesthetic sensations in addition to pain and temperature, confirming earlier clinical reports of autopsied cases and adding to the evidence that thermal and nociceptive information was distributed among brain structures with functions that were not limited to pain. Some of the patients with thalamic lesions, most often caused by a stroke, also developed constant pain within the area of impaired pain sensation (a central pain syndrome), again confirming earlier autopsy-based reports and suggesting that the lesion had interrupted an endogenous sensory control mechanism. CT scanning also showed that lesions within different and widely separated regions of the cerebral cortex could affect pain. Damage of the white matter below the insular and secondary somatic sensory cortices (S2) impaired tactile and thermal sensations in addition to pain and, like some lesions in the thalamus, also produced a central pain syndrome similar to that associated with thalamic lesions. CT scans of surgical patients with chronic pain confirmed that surgical lesions within the midline cingulate cortex (see Figure 4.1) of the limbic system, a cortical area distinct from the somatic sensory areas (S1 cortex), produced impaired attention in addition to reducing the negative hedonic or affective component of pain. The perceived chronic pain intensity, however, was only mildly affected, if at all.

The development and implementation of magnetic resonance imaging (MRI)[4] enhanced the anatomical resolution of brain imaging and has since dominated the analysis of CNS lesions. The results[5] have confirmed the earlier observations that CNS lesions affecting pain (1) also affect other somatic sensory functions, (2) may produce a central pain syndrome combined (paradoxically) with an attenuation of evoked pain, and (3) are distributed among several cortical and subcortical sites.

An unusual clinical case also provided evidence for the anatomically parallel processing of affective and sensory discriminative components of pain.[6] In a patient with profoundly impaired tactile, kinesthetic, and thermal sensations in one hand, MRI revealed a lesion confined to the primary (S1) and secondary (S2) somatosensory areas of the opposite postcentral gyrus of the cerebral cortex. Noxious heat stimulation of the involved hand at more than twice the pain threshold for the normal hand failed to evoke any pain and instead evoked a feeling of marked unpleasantness emanating vaguely from the arm area. Thus, the parallel distribution of nociceptive information allows an isolated negative hedonic experience to emerge alone, unaccompanied by the physical, temporal, and detailed spatial information normally provided by the somatosensory cortex of the parietal lobe. Anatomical-clinical correlation studies like those cited here challenge a simple phrenological model of pain mechanisms by showing that nociceptive information is distributed to brain areas that participate in sensory and neurological functions other than pain, and that some of these pathways act in parallel to mediate the discriminative and affective components of pain.[7]

In summary, anatomical imaging of the living human brain, combined with quantitative sensory testing and clinical information, instantiates and amplifies three main concepts that form a basis for a conceptual model of pain: (1) nociceptive information is *distributed* among anatomically and functionally distinct CNS structures that collectively create pain, (2) pain is *modulated* by anatomically, physiologically, and functionally distinct circuits throughout the CNS, and (3) nociceptive activity itself triggers *endogenous feedback* mechanisms that affect the perception of pain. But where and when is all this neural activity taking place? What does the circuitry look like? And how can it be measured? To address these questions, we need not only to see the brain but also to see the activity, how much there is, and where it is occurring.

THE DEVELOPMENT OF FUNCTIONAL IMAGING

Functional imaging is a major advance in neuroscience because it enables a real-time correlation of localized CNS activity with a specific function. As considered here, functional imaging allows an assessment of the activity of *all* anatomically visible cortical and subcortical parts of the CNS during the performance of specific tasks. The "task" might be very simple, such as wiggling a finger, or very complex, like performing a calculation or rating the hedonic quality of a painless or painful stimulus. "Parts of the CNS" are made visible by using MRI or CT. Electroencephalography (EEG), magnetoencephalography (MEG), or evoked potential methods that are limited to the cerebral cortex are excluded by the definition of imaging used here. Optical imaging,[8] which uses voltage-sensitive dyes, changes in blood oxygenation, or changes in the biophysical properties of cell membranes, will also not be discussed in detail here because, although very useful for investigating the activity of localized neuronal populations, it is limited to small, exposed surfaces and cannot assess the conjoint activation of multiple functionally related areas throughout the CNS. The brain is the most frequent target for functional imaging, but the brainstem and spinal cord can be imaged also.

The "assessment of activity" is the tricky part of functional imaging. The activity of interest, of course, is that of neurons; however, depending on what is being measured, the activity of glial cells may variably contribute to activity estimates also. Thus far, "activity" has meant changes in the voltage measured across neuronal membranes; these are the action or synaptic potentials. It is now possible, however, to use magnetic resonance spectroscopy (MRS),[9] together with anatomical imaging (MRI), to reveal selected features of the chemical composition of different brain areas during different experimental and clinical conditions. Another measure of activity, to be discussed later, is positron emission tomography (PET), which enables an estimate of a neurotransmitter's binding to its receptor.

It is not possible to obtain these electrical or chemical measurements for each neuron within large groups of cells distributed among different structures like the cerebral cortex, thalamus, and brainstem. To obtain an estimate of the activity of groups of neurons, we must be content with a surrogate measure of activity within the CNS. The surrogate measure that has emerged is an increase in regional cerebral blood flow (rCBF) and an electromagnetic signal (discussed later) that accompanies it.

In 1890, Sir Charles Sherrington and his colleague, C. S. Roy, published their evidence that, in the anesthetized mammal, cerebral blood volume increased following electrical stimulation of a sensory nerve.[10] They showed that this increase in blood volume could be produced by the intravenous injection of an extract of mammalian brain tissue and concluded that the sensory nerve stimulation produced cerebral metabolic changes that increased blood flow to the entire brain. Since then, neurosurgeons have observed, usually through a dissecting microscope, *localized* increases in blood perfusion in the exposed cerebral cortex of conscious patients instructed to perform a simple task during surgical operations.[11] These early observations indicated that the increased blood flow was not simply a global response of the entire brain but was at least partially restricted to localized areas of increased neuronal activity. However, the link between neuronal activity and rCBF was not seriously investigated for many years. In fact, the quantitative and temporal relationship between the two has been determined only within the past two decades, largely because of technical advances.

SOME ESSENTIAL BACKGROUND

Bear with me here for the next several paragraphs because the interpretation of functional imaging studies, including studies of pain, requires at least some knowledge of what is being measured, how the studies are conducted, and how they may be interpreted.

The Hemodynamic Response

The blood flow changes during local neuronal activity constitute the hemodynamic response (HDR), a critical part of functional imaging because it is the proximate cause of the change in rCBF that, in turn, is the surrogate estimate of the activity of spatially localized groups of neurons. What exactly triggers the hemodynamic response is uncertain. There is evidence that neurotransmitter release activates a calcium-mediated release of vasodilatory metabolites by astrocytic glial cells appended to blood vessels.[12] And there is no doubt that, within the important limitations discussed later, the HDR is driven by local neuroelectrical activity and metabolic demand. Therefore, to interpret functional imaging studies correctly, we need to have some understanding of the HDR and how it is related to measures of neuronal activity.

The temporal dynamics of the HDR are shown at the *top* in Figure 9.1. As detected by wavelength-specific optical imaging of the surface of a rat's cerebral cortex, a brief sensory (facial whisker) stimulus (about one second) evokes neuronal synaptic and action potential activity (spiking). This neuronal activity immediately increases oxygen consumption and reduces the local concentration of oxygenated blood hemoglobin (oxyhemoglobin, or HbO); this is the "initial dip" in HbO shown at the top of Figure 9.1. At the same time, the concentration of deoxygenated blood hemoglobin (HbD) increases. This period of deoxygenation is followed, within 1 to 2 seconds, by a marked inflow of oxygenated blood, which peaks in about 4 seconds and recovers about 2 seconds after peaking; this period is the "overshoot" in Figure 9.1. It is called an overshoot because measurements of local oxygen and glucose consumption show that the increased volume of oxygenated blood exceeds the local metabolic demand for oxygen.[13] The duration of the oxygenation inflow period can be extended by simply increasing the duration of neuronal activity. In most studies, a small, transient after-period of reduced oxygenated blood (an "undershoot") can be seen, but this is of uncertain significance and will not be discussed further. As shown in Figure 9.1, the HDR is a sluggish, delayed, and exaggerated indicator of neuronal activity, at least as measured most accurately by the optical imaging of hemoglobin oxygenation changes in rat somatosensory cortex. In addition to its temporal sluggishness, the HDR overrepresents the amount of neuronal spiking and synaptic activity at the higher end of neuronal response intensity.

Optical imaging experiments show that the minimal evoked hemodynamic response covers an area that far exceeds the 0.121-mm^2 cross section of a rat whisker column (5.6 mm^2 during early deoxygenation, increasing to about 20 mm^2 during the later oxygenation phase). This spatial spread of the HDR occupies an area *167 times larger* than the cross-sectional area of the column responsible for its generation. Of course, the spatial distribution of the HDR is determined by the microanatomy of the blood capillaries. But assuming that the HDR shown here is due only to the activity of neurons in a single whisker column, it nonetheless would represent 22,500 action potentials generated by the approximately 18,000 neurons in that column during that one-second, 5-Hz stimulus. The area occupied by the HDR suggests that neuronal spiking and subthreshold synaptic activity in neighboring whisker columns could contribute to the HDR. These estimates show that, with minimal sensory stimulation, a small hemodynamic response probably represents the activity of far more than 10,000 neurons and greatly exceeds the spatial extent of the presumed active area.[14] The contribution of glial cell energy demands to the HDR is unknown.

This HDR estimate of total neuronal activity is based on excitatory synaptic activity; it does not provide an estimate of the inhibitory synaptic activity generated by

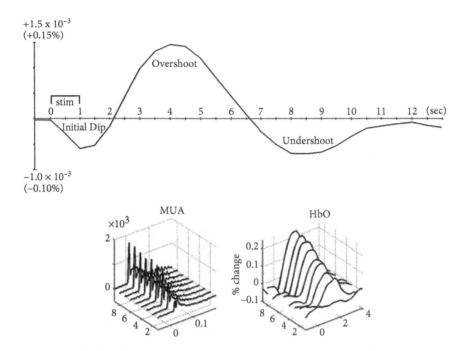

FIGURE 9.1. The hemodynamic response and neuronal activity in a rat cortical whisker column. (Note that Neurons of the higher mammalian sensory cortices [somatic, visual, auditory] are arranged in vertical columns and six horizontal layers. Neurons within each column generate action potentials in response to similar types of stimuli delivered within similar locations of the sensory field [body surface, visual space, auditory pitch]. Within the somatosensory cortex, for example, one column might respond to movement of hair and another to movement of a joint; but no one has found a column for pain. See: Mountcastle VB. The columnar organization of the neocortex. *Brain 120*: 701–722, 1997.) The measurements are made over a cortical column of neurons excited only by that particular whisker. *Top*: Time course of the hemodynamic response (HDR). The concentration of oxygenated hemoglobin (HbO) at the surface of rat somatosensory cortex is measured over time (0–13 seconds) as a percentage change from the level just before wiggling a rat's whisker (at 5 Hz) for one second. *Bottom left*: The action potential activity of multiple neurons (multiple unit activity, or MUA) within a single rat whisker column is measured (vertical "y" axis in spikes/sec) over time (horizontal "x" axis, 0–0.1-0.2 sec) following multiple single whisker movements at increasing relative amplitudes ("z" axis, 28). *Bottom right*: The percentage change in HbO is measured (vertical "y" axis) over the same whisker column following the different whisker stimulation intensities shown at the left. Note that the time ("x") axis is here displayed as 04 seconds, not in tenths of seconds as in the measure of MUA. Note that (1) the period of neuronal spiking begins and ends well before the onset of the HDR, (2) the HDR peaks and decays long after neuronal spiking has ceased, and (3) the neuronal spiking response reaches a maximum (by stimulus intensity ~5) while the HDR response continues to increase. The results are similar if electrophysiological measurements of synaptic, rather than just spiking, activity are used (the local field potential or LFP).

Data at *top* from Chen-Bee CH, Agoncillo T, Xiong Y, and Frostig RD. The triphasic intrinsic signal: implications for functional imaging. *Journal of Neuroscience 27*: 4572–4586, 2007, with permission of the Society for Neuroscience; data at *bottom* from Devor A, Dunn AK, Andermann ML, Ulbert I, Boas DA, and Dale AM. Coupling of total hemoglobin concentration, oxygenation, and neural activity in rat somatosensory cortex. *Neuron 39*: 353–359, 2003, with permission of Elsevier; Devor A, Ulbert I, Dunn AK, Narayanan SN, Jones SR, Andermann ML, Boas DA, and Dale AM. Coupling of the cortical hemodynamic response to cortical and thalamic neuronal activity. *Proceedings of the National Academy of Sciences USA 102*: 3822–3827, 2005. See also: Sheth SA, Nemoto M, Guiou M, Walker M, Pouratian N, and Toga AW. Linear and nonlinear relationships between neuronal activity, oxygen metabolism, and hemodynamic responses. *Neuron 42*: 347–355, 2004.

neurons generating inhibitory synaptic potentials (IPSPs; see section on the neuron in the Appendix). In fact, direct recording experiments in animal models show that synaptic activity, not action potential generation or spiking, is likely the primary contributor to the HDR and that the HDR reflects both inhibitory and excitatory synaptic activity.[15] Therefore, changes in rCBF should be interpreted as changes in the intensity of synaptic activity generally, not simply as changes in excitatory synaptic transmission. Within a synaptically active region, however, the predominant synaptic effect is likely to be excitatory because the inhibitory neurons are generally short-axoned cells (interneurons) within a local circuit and are themselves activated by excitatory synapses from outside the local circuit.

In summary, the HDR reflects the activity of neurons but, as might be expected of any surrogate measurement, it is an imperfect estimate. Its spatial distribution is at least partly determined by microvascular anatomy. The "activity" represented by the HDR appears to be a mixture of neuronal action and synaptic potentials (predominantly the latter). However, although the synaptic activity predominantly excites neurons, an unknown proportion of synaptic activity is inhibitory, and the HDR is blind to this distinction. The number of neurons needed to generate an HDR is unknown, but evidence from several experiments suggests that the number is in the range of at least tens of thousands. More intense and prolonged stimuli, such as those used in human imaging studies, evoke neuronal (and glial) activity and HDRs that are very much larger. The HDR lags behind and extends beyond neuronal activity by about 2 seconds and continues to increase after neuronal activity has reached a plateau. The oxygen delivered by the HDR exceeds the oxygen used by local neuronal activity but appears to supply the glucose required for combined neuronal and glial activity during synaptic transmission. Nonetheless, within these limitations, noninvasive measurements of rCBF give us an opportunity to estimate the location, timing, and intensity of the activity of neurons in the CNS of awake humans.

Functional Imaging: Functional Magnetic Resonance Imaging and Positron Emission Tomography

Functional imaging is certainly not focused on the neurophysiology of rat whisker columns. As used in studies of humans, the stimulus (or task) excites more neurons and is more prolonged. The HDRs are therefore generated over a much more extensive volume of CNS tissue, resulting in more prolonged rCBF and tissue perfusion.

Most functional imaging studies today are performed using MRI, called functional MRI (fMRI).[16] This method takes advantage of the different magnetic properties of HbO and HbD during the HDR. Because the images are acquired within a large magnetic field (the scanner), an electromagnetic signal is emitted when the axial orientation of hydrogen nuclei (protons) is displaced and recovers from repetitive electromagnetic pulses introduced into the scanner. The signal is affected by the different magnetic properties of HbO and HbD. HbD, which is slightly magnetic, is increased during the early HDR (the "initial dip" at the top of Figure 9.1); this interferes with the electromagnetic signal generated by protons. But HbO, which is magnetically neutral, replaces the HbD and is markedly increased during the highly oxygenated "overshoot" period, thus allowing the full electromagnetic signal to be detected. The signal is therefore called the blood-oxygen-level dependent (BOLD) signal, and it is present throughout the overshoot period of the HDR and therefore throughout the period of neuronal synaptic activity. Of course, because the HDR is slower than the neuronal activity, the BOLD signal is slightly delayed and prolonged (Figure 9.2).

Nonetheless, it is clear that the BOLD signal provides a reasonably good estimate of the magnitude and duration of neuronal activity. As noted previously, however, the synaptic activity detected with fMRI is a mixture of excitation and inhibition with excitatory activity predominating. Therefore, changes in the amplitude of the BOLD signal are best interpreted as increases or decreases in excitation, keeping in mind that inhibitory neurons within the local circuitry may be the targets of this excitation.

The ability of anatomical MRI to reveal the basic anatomy of CNS pathways and neuronal assemblies deep within the brain, brainstem, and even the spinal cord allows

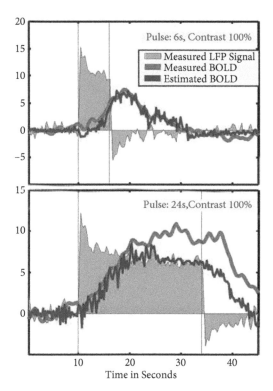

FIGURE 9.2. Temporal and intensity relationship of the measured (*blue*) and modeled (*red*) BOLD response with neuronal activity (*gray area*) evoked in the visual cerebral cortex of an anesthetized monkey during visual stimulation of different durations. Neural activity is recorded as the local field potential (LFP), which represents primarily synaptic activity. The signal amplitudes, relative to prestimulus baseline, are shown on the vertical axis. On the scales for this figure, the "initial dip" and the delay of the BOLD signal with respect to neuronal activity are not seen. The delay of the BOLD offset following the end of neuronal activity is obvious.

From Logothetis NK. The underpinnings of the BOLD functional magnetic resonance imaging signal. *Journal of Neuroscience 23*: 3963–3971, 2003, with permission of the Society for Neuroscience.

us also to locate the source of activity. But what is the detailed spatiotemporal pattern of this activity and how localized is it? How many neurons are represented by the BOLD response, which is derived from the HDR? As noted earlier, the very small HDR studied by exciting one column of neurons in the rat's whisker cortex represents the activity of tens of thousands of neurons, and probably many more. The spatial resolution of fMRI is much less and is determined by the technical limitations of the scanner and by the image acquisition choices of the experimenter. The unit of resolution is a three-dimensional pixel, called a *voxel*. According to one estimate, the average voxel in a typical MRI study is about 55 mm^3 (~ 3.8 mm on each side of a cube) and contains about 5.5 million neurons and about 20 to 50 billion synapses. Another source estimates that there are 630,000 neurons in a slightly smaller voxel.[17] For comparison, consider that the "brain" (mushroom body) volume of the common housefly is only 0.3 mm^3 and contains an estimated 338,000 neurons; the estimate is similar for other insects[18] (summarized in Table 9.1). Given the complex sensory functions and extensive behavioral repertoire of insects generally, it seems safe to conclude that, depending on circuit architecture, highly complex neuronal computations could be occurring within one voxel of an fMRI scan. And each of the several sites of activation detected in a typical human fMRI scan is comprised of multiple voxels, often hundreds or thousands. This means that each site of activation detected in an fMRI voxel could represent multiple different complex patterns of neuronal activity and functions rather than a single, homogeneous function, as is often assumed when interpreting fMRI or other functional imaging studies. Think of a satellite view of North America at night; the distribution of light density tells you that Los Angelis and New York City are far more active than Kansas City, but the details of these activities and how they differ are unknown.

There is an additional limitation of fMRI (and PET) that arises from the need to decide which of thousands or hundreds of thousands of potentially active voxels in the brain are activated by a condition of interest, like pain, and which should be considered background noise, reflecting the activity of neurons engaged in nonpain functions, like maintaining wakefulness or attention. This problem is addressed by employing powerful statistical analysis programs to the analysis of imaging data. To avoid the inclusion of "noise" voxels, the threshold for detecting condition-related voxel activity is usually selected to favor noise exclusion and thus avoid false-positive detection.[19] This means that, like a topographical map of earth's terrain, functional brain imaging is blind to potentially important information that may lie below the peaks. Nonetheless, with the previous limitations in mind, functional imaging provides important information about

Table 9.1. Estimated Number of Neurons in Functional Magnetic Resonance Imaging Voxels and in the Brain (Mushroom Body) of an Insect*

Structure	Size (mm^3)	No. of Neurons
MRI voxel1	55 (3.8 mm/side)	5×10^6
MRI voxel2	27 (3.0 mm/side)	0.63×10^6
Fly brain	0.34 (0.7 mm/side)	0.34×10^6

*See text for discussion and references.

the location and intensity of neuronal activity during specified behaviors, including the perception of pain.

Some functional imaging studies, such as PET, tag the blood by intravenously injecting a mildly radioactive molecule or compound. For example, a modified radioactive form of glucose is temporarily trapped inside neurons in approximate proportion to their combined neuroelectrical and metabolic activity, thus allowing surrounding detectors in a scanner to locate, in three dimensions, neurons that are more metabolically active than comparison neurons elsewhere in the CNS.[20] This method is widely used for clinical imaging today. The size of PET voxels, however, is larger than for fMRI, so the spatial resolution is less. To detect localized changes in rCBF, slightly radioactive water is injected instead of radioactive glucose.[21] This method of detecting transient brain activation does not require the detection of BOLD electromagnetic signals and has the advantage of providing a baseline condition that is more temporally stable than in fMRI. Another method that is focused on detecting rCBF changes is arterial spin labeling (ASL).[22] Arterial blood flowing to the brain volume of interest is "tagged" with a radiofrequency pulse (displacing protons), and the electromagnetic signal generated (as the protons recover) during the HDR is contrasted with the null signal in an adjacent unresponsive volume. ASL has the advantage of detecting arterial (oxygenated) blood more directly and specifically than conventional fMRI, thus avoiding that fraction of the signal generated by venous blood draining an inactive region. As ASL technology advances, this method is likely to be used more frequently in functional brain imaging studies.

PET can also be used to determine whether a neurotransmitter such as an endogenous opioid or dopamine has been released at a specific location.[23] A slightly radioactive synthetic compound that binds to the same postsynaptic receptors as the neurotransmitter is injected intravenously as a "probe." The fraction of the injected compound that has bonded with the receptors can be determined by periodically sampling the blood. If the endogenous neurotransmitter has been released during the injection period, a smaller than expected fraction of the injected probe compound will bond with the receptor, giving an estimate of the change in the amount of binding due to neurotransmitter release.

Voxel-Based Morphometry

Finally, it has now become possible to use voxel-based-morphometry (VBM) to assess the volume of gray matter in MRI studies.[24] This is possible because MRI is able to distinguish easily the difference between the neuronal-containing gray matter and the myelin-containing white matter of the brain. VBM can be used to detect changes in gray matter volume across time and between groups of subjects. Gray matter changes detected by VBM cannot identify the cellular elements responsible for the volume change. It cannot be assumed that changes in neuronal or synaptic number or size alone cause VBM changes because glial cells, for example, could contribute to the observed effect. Nonetheless, it has been used to assess long-term changes attributable to chronic, persistent pain, as discussed next in Chapter 10.

10

FUNCTIONAL IMAGING CONTRIBUTIONS
TO CHASING PAIN

Given the foregoing background for understanding and evaluating functional imaging studies, I offer a personally selected sample of contributions from among the many "pain imaging" studies that have been performed over the last approximately two and a half decades. A recent meta-analysis of functional brain imaging studies of pain among healthy persons and patients revealed 170 peer-reviewed papers published during the years 1990 through 2014.[1] My quick MEDLINE searches (pain + brain + fMRI + human) and (pain + brain + positron emission tomography + human) identified 50 functional magnetic resonance imaging (fMRI) and 21 positron emission tomography (PET) studies published since 2014 (through 2017). I will not risk getting lost in that forest of approximately 241 papers, so here is my personal take on the highlights.

THE DEFAULT STATE OF THE BRAIN

As noted in the Appendix, the brain is silent only in death. Electroencephalography (EEG) recordings for many years have shown us that there is plenty of neuronal activity during sleep and that this activity changes dramatically during the various stages of sleep, especially during dreaming. Because we are interested in comparing brain activity during pain-free and painful states during wakefulness, it is necessary to establish a brain condition or "state" that could reasonably be considered "task free" but awake.[2] You might imagine that, in this resting state, brain metabolism would be low compared with that during the performance of a difficult cognitive task or experiencing pain. Not so. The brain is a very expensive organ from a metabolic point of view—and the metabolic demands continue while resting and awake, eyes open or closed, doing nothing. It has been estimated that the brain is only 2% of average adult body weight but accounts for nearly 20% of total body metabolism at rest. As noted in the Appendix, approximately 80% of this energy is required for recycling neurotransmitters released during synaptic activity and for maintaining the resting electrical charge across neuronal membranes. In terms of blood flow, our three-pound resting adult brain (whether you weigh 90 or 300 pounds) takes up nearly 15% of the total blood output of the heart each minute.[3] But the increased regional cerebral blood flow (rCBF) observed during functional imaging studies amounts to no more than 5% of the total brain blood flow (global cerebral blood flow [CBF] is ~700 mL/minute). Thus, the metabolic cost of cognitive tasks or the experience of severe pain is small compared with the cost of maintaining a resting brain. So, what is the brain doing during wakeful resting and why is this important for the functional imaging of the brain during pain?

During wakeful, task-free resting, the blood flow to the brain is not distributed evenly. Studies performed on healthy adult volunteers (ages 19 to 84 years) show that the midline (medial) surface of the cerebral cortex—extending from the tip of the frontal lobe, throughout the cingulate (limbic) gyrus, to the beginning of the visual cortex, including multisensory integrating areas of the lateral parietal lobe—has much greater blood flow, and hence more metabolic activity, than the rest of the brain during wakeful resting (Figure 10.1). Because CBF is distributed largely according to the metabolic demands of synaptic maintenance, the uneven distribution of CBF suggests that these limbic and parietal cortical areas remain as though in a state of protective vigilance, ready to detect external or internal events that could affect the individual's survival.

Perhaps some of the resting activity could be attributed to the ongoing resting activity of the small-diameter nerve fibers in sensory nerves.[4] In support of this "sentinel" hypothesis, these cortical areas become *deactivated*, showing a reduction of rCBF as the individual moves from the resting state to one of alert engagement with various tasks. In effect, the surveillance-alarm system has been deactivated so that neuronal resources and brain activity can be distributed elsewhere.

Of particular relevance for understanding pain neurobiology, these areas, especially the medial prefrontal and cingulate cortex, are *activated*, showing increased rCBF during pain, as will be discussed in subsequent paragraphs. How can this be? One might imagine that the compelling experience of pain would call forth even greater deactivation than engaging in a cognitively demanding task, for example. An explanation for this apparent paradox is provided by combined behavioral and functional PET experiments[5] showing

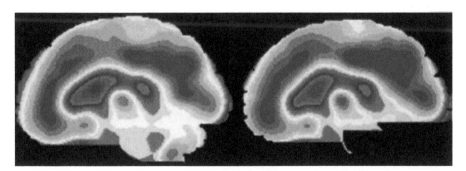

FIGURE 10.1. Color-coded images of blood flow to the midline (i.e., medial) surfaces of the left (reader's left) and right hemispheres during wakeful resting with eyes closed. The images are about 3 to 5 millimeters to the left or right of the fissure separating the hemispheres. In each image, the frontal lobe is to the far left and the occipital lobe is to the right. The thalamus and upper brainstem protrude upward into the fluid-filled ventricle (*blue*) of each hemisphere. The greatest blood flow (*red*) extends from the medial frontal lobe throughout the cingulate gyrus, forming a ring (limbus) around the thalamus and upper brainstem. Not shown here is the relatively increased blood flow in some sensory integrating areas of the parietal cortex of the outer (lateral) surface of each hemisphere.

(Excerpted from Raichle ME, MacLeod AM, Snyder AZ, Powers WJ, Gusnard, Da, and Shulman GL. A default mode of brain function. *Proceedings of the National Academy of Science USA 98*: 676–682, with permission of The National Academy of Science, USA.)

that these cortical areas, together with the hypothalamus and central gray matter of the upper brainstem, are either less deactivated or actually activated during *anxiety*. Thus, the emotional experience of anxiety overrides the underlying deactivation process, resulting in increased, rather than decreased, rCBF in these brain areas. Perhaps different neurons or different patterns of neuronal activity within these anatomical regions are involved here; we cannot tell because of the limited spatial resolution of functional imaging discussed earlier. Linking the previous observations to pain requires the reasonable assumption that the aversive emotional, negative hedonic experiences common to anxiety, fear, and pain are subjectively and biologically similar although not identical. Note that these experiments suggest again that brain structures identified nearly 80 years ago by James Papez, and later conceptually united as a limbic system, appear to be critical participants in, or even mediators of, emotional experience.[6] PET activation studies of self-induced emotion reveal activity in the cingulate, insular, and somatosensory cortices as well as the hypothalamus, adding further support for the association of limbic system structures to emotional experience.[7]

PAIN EMERGES FROM THE CONJOINT ACTIVATION OF STRUCTURES MEDIATING SENSORY, AFFECTIVE, AND COGNITIVE FUNCTIONS

Early PET studies showed that the somatosensory (S1, S2), limbic (cingulate, insula) cortices, lateral and medial thalamus, and upper brainstem (including periaqueductal gray, or PAG), were active specifically during pain and did not simply reflect the detection of differences in stimulus intensity. Changes in perceived intensity were reflected in the responses of both somatosensory and limbic structures, consistent with their conjoint participation in creating pain.[8] Later, using hypnosis, it was possible to modify selectively the perception of the unpleasantness of a painful stimulus, thus uncoupling it from the affectively neutral perception of stimulus intensity, and reveal that cingulate cortex activation is correlated with the degree of unpleasantness while the activation of the primary somatosensory cortex (S1) is not (Figure 10.2).[9] Another way of examining the link between limbic structures and the negative affect of pain is to observe the brain activation pattern during *allodynia*, the experience of exaggerated unpleasantness during normally painless stimulation of injured or sensitized skin (think of touching a sunburn). As expected, after controlling for stimulus intensity, the unpleasantness of allodynia is strongly associated with the activation of structures and pathways making up the limbic system (e.g., cingulate and orbital prefrontal cortices, medial thalamus).[10] Subsequent magnetoencephalography (MEG) studies show that limbic and somatosensory cortices are activated in close temporal contiguity; in fact, a recent intracerebral recording study of patients undergoing testing before surgery for epilepsy revealed that several cortical limbic, sensory, and motor areas are activated *simultaneously* immediately before the reaction (in ~350 milliseconds) to a painful laser stimulus.[11]

Many subsequent PET and fMRI studies confirm that an assembly of brain structures consisting of a "core membership" and "frequently affiliated members" (my phrases) is activated during pain (Figure 10.3).[12] The core members are those that are regularly activated in most pain neuroimaging studies and include the anterior cingulate cortex, the

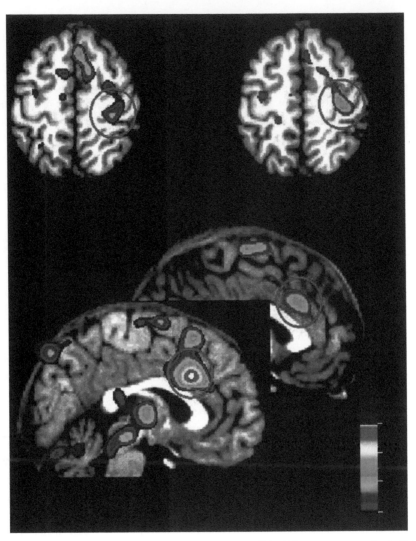

FIGURE 10.2. Color-coded statistical map of regional cerebral blood flow responses to identically intense noxious heat stimuli perceived, under hypnosis, as either highly unpleasant (*left* images) or not
unpleasant (*right* images). Color bar at *lower right* indicates high (*red*) or low (*blue-violet*) statistical
significance of the response. *Upper* images of the top cortical surface show statistically insignificant
responses in the primary (S1) somatosensory cortex during both high (*left*) and low (*right*) perceived
unpleasantness. *Lower* images of the medial (inner) surface of the left hemisphere show highly significant responses in the anterior cingulate cortex only during the highly unpleasant condition (*left*).
(From Rainville P, Duncan GH, Price DD, Carrier M, and Bushnell MC. Pain affect encoded in human anterior
cingulate but not somatosensory cortex. *Science 277*: 968–971, 1997, with permission of the American Association
for the Advancement of Science.)

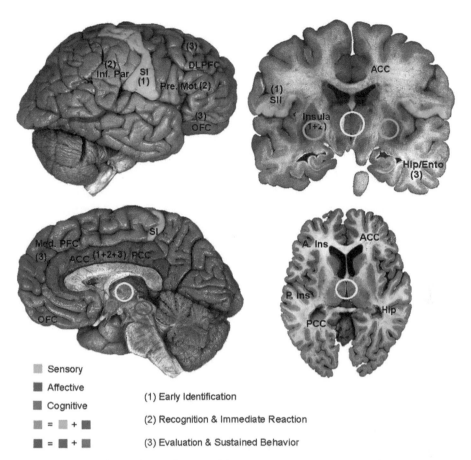

Sensory
Affective
Cognitive

■ = ■ + ■

■ = ■ + ■

(1) Early Identification

(2) Recognition & Immediate Reaction

(3) Evaluation & Sustained Behavior

FIGURE 10.3. Sites that are frequently activated during positron emission tomography or functional magnetic resonance imaging studies of pain. Brain images are shown in lateral (*upper left*), coronal (*upper right*), medial or sagittal (*lower left*), and horizontal (*lower right*) views. The figure depicts cortical areas in colors that indicate their hypothesized participation in the principal components of pain according to the inserted legend. The numbers indicate their hypothesized pain-related functions in the temporal domain. Commonly activated subcortical structures are indicated by *circles*: thalamus (*yellow*), basal ganglia (*green*), hypothalamus (*orange*), and upper brainstem and periaqueductal gray (*blue*). The cerebellum, which has strong connections with the frontal lobe, is between the brainstem and occipital (posterior) lobe of the brain. *A*, anterior; *CC*, cingulate cortex; *DLPFC*, dorsolateral prefrontal cortex; *Ento*, entorhinal cortex; *Hip*, hippocampus; *Inf*, inferior; *Ins*, insula; *Med PFC*, medial prefrontal cortex; *OFC*, orbitofrontal cortex; *P*, posterior; *Par*, parietal; *Pre Mot*, premotor; *S*, somatosensory (I and II).

Adapted from Figure 3 in Casey KL, and Tran TD. Cortical mechanisms mediating acute and chronic pain in humans. In: Cervero F, and Jensen TS (Eds.), *Pain, Handbook of Clinical Neurology*, Volume 81, Chapter 12. Edinburgh: Elsevier, 2006, pp. 159–177.

insular cortex, the somatosensory cortices (S1, S2, or both), and the thalamus (medial or ventrolateral). The affiliated members are very often, but less frequently, activated during pain and include components of the basal ganglia, upper brainstem (area of the PAG), hypothalamus, orbitofrontal cortex, medial prefrontal cortex, and cerebellum. There is strong evidence that a heat pain activation pattern developed from a large population of healthy participants is specific for physical and not purely emotional pain or distress, and that the magnitude of the responses of some structures, such as the ventrolateral thalamus and the S1 and S2 somatosensory cortices, signals stimulus location rather than unpleasantness or affect.[13] Taken together, the results give neurophysiological substance to the conceptual model of pain and the International Association for the Study of Pain definition of pain as the conjoint activity of affective and sensory mechanisms in the brain.[14]

More Caveats: The Salience Network

Before concluding that the pattern of activity shown in Figure 10.3 ends the chase for pain, we must recall the limitations of functional imaging as discussed in Chapter 9 (see the section on "Some Essential Background") and add some additional caveats. Although an fMRI study has identified an activation pattern or "signature" of physical pain as distinct from warmth or from emotional or social "pain,"[15] there remains the possibility that many of these structures also mediate other functions and are not strictly specific for physical pain. There is evidence, for example, that structures such as the cingulate, insular, and orbitofrontal cortices and the inner (or middle) parts of the thalamus receive painless somatosensory, auditory, visual, and other sensory information. The BOLD responses in some of these structures appear to be determined by how well these sensory inputs are perceived to stand out from background or "noisy" sensations, a property called *salience*. According to this interpretation, the structures activated during pain are part of a "salience network" (Figure 10.4) that has a direct pathway from the thalamus to the limbic cortex and to related autonomic and motor mechanisms for defensive behavior.[16]

A statistical conjunction analysis identifies the structures activated by each novel stimulus of each sensory modality. This shows that many structures activated by noxious stimuli (parietal operculum, insula, posterior parietal cortex, anterior cingulate cortex) are also activated by novel innocuous stimuli. Tactile somatosensory and noxious stimuli that are outside this salience network are shown in blue and red, respectively.

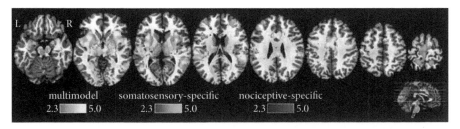

FIGURE 10.4. Functional magnetic resonance imaging study revealing a salience network (*yellow*) activated by brief visual, auditory, tactile, or noxious somatic stimuli presented in a random sequence to emphasize stimulus novelty.
From Legrain V, Iannetti GD, Plaghki L, and Mouraux A. The pain matrix reloaded A salience detection system for the body. *Progress in Neurobiology 93*: 111–124, 2011, with permission from Elsevier.

The activation of somatosensory structures such as the S2 cortex and the somatosensory thalamus would seem to tie this group of activations to physical pain rather than to some generalized salience. However, somatosensory, thalamic, and limbic structures are also activated in neuroimaging studies of spider phobias, for example.[17] Noxious somatic and visceral stimuli could certainly excite this network, especially the somatosensory cortex and thalamus, more effectively than many other sensory inputs, but this group of structures, according to the "salience" argument, would not be considered a "pain network" exclusively. Additional support for this argument comes from the observation that many "pain-activated" structures are activated by novel noxious somatic stimuli presented to individuals who are genetically painless (see Chapter 7, section on "Genetics and Ion Channels").[18] Rather, pain could be considered as emerging from activity *within* the salience mechanism when it is excited by input from nociceptors. This means that the neurons with activity that is essential for the unique, unified experience of pain are somewhere within the salience network, perhaps hidden beneath and among the activation peaks detected by fMRI methods. The application of automated, large-scale, multivariate meta-analysis can help associate specific brain activation patterns with unique cognitive states and experiences like pain.[19] But, even among the active voxels, the hundreds of thousands, or even millions, of neurons within a typical voxel or cluster of voxels allows enough variation of response among voxels to add undetected complexity and functional flexibility to the network detected by fMRI (see Table 9.1).

Another way of assessing the meaning of the activation pattern during pain is to recall the effect of destructive lesions. We have seen, for example, that focal lesions do not simply attenuate pain; they may also impair tactile abilities and cognitive functions. They may impair the ability to localize pain while leaving intact its negative hedonic component. The reverse condition, namely, intact somatosensory function with emotional or cognitive deficits, may follow lesions within limbic structures such as the cingulate cortex. In addition, lesions within the somatosensory thalamus or cortex may cause, rather than relieve, pain (the central pain syndromes). In short, it is very difficult, if not impossible, to completely and selectively eliminate pain (and retain consciousness) with a focal lesion in the CNS, including lesions within these pain-activated structures. Even if there is temporary pain relief, the capacity of the CNS to at least partially reorganize neuronal networks leads to a return of pain or other equally unpleasant somatic sensations.

Finally, it is important to consider that the activation of structures identified in functional imaging studies does not necessarily tie that activation to a single function (however defined). As noted previously, there are abundant neuronal resources within one or a few voxels to support a wide, although necessarily limited, repertoire of functions (see Table 9.1). There is strong evidence, for example, that pain-activated structures, including those within the commonly defined limbic system, may be activated also during *positively hedonic* experiences such as the *relief* from pain.

Thus, the perceived intensity of noxious heat stimulation can be greatly reduced immediately after terminating the noxious stimulus, a phenomenon called "offset analgesia" (OA). During OA, there is an activation of brainstem and cerebral structures that are also activated during evoked pain, showing that these structures (including the cerebellum!!) participate in both the bottom-up excitation and top-down suppression of pain and pain-related behavior.[20] These observations emphasize the need for caution in interpreting the functional significance of the responses seen in functional imaging studies.[21]

Although the current identity of pain-activated structures is critically important for a useful conceptual model of pain, our level of confidence in its verity and utility must be constrained by the considerations discussed previously and by the technical limitations of functional brain imaging. Also keep in mind that functional imaging, as currently implemented, is focused primarily on the cerebral (and cerebellar) cortex and reveals much less about the activity in smaller groups of neurons in subcortical structures; this will be considered further in Chapter 11.

THE COGNITIVE MODULATION OF PAIN

The *placebo*[22] effect, an enhancement of treatment by suggestion or expectation, is perhaps the most frequently referenced cognitive process associated with pain relief. The magnitude of the placebo effect varies considerably among individuals and depends on the means used to evoke it, but overall it is sufficiently strong to require a placebo control group in clinical trials of new analgesics and of many other drugs. For example, a large clinical trial of acupuncture for common musculoskeletal low back pain shows that both sham (placebo) and true acupuncture are equally effective in providing clinically significant pain relief compared with conventional physiotherapy and drug treatment.[23] The *nocebo* effect is the opposite of the placebo; it is produced by the suggestion of treatment failure or, in the case of pain, hyperalgesia. In fact, these suggestions may be effective even if not consciously perceived! Simple verbal suggestion, however, is less effective than the manipulation of expectations by deceptive conditioning. For example, an experimenter can covertly reduce or increase the intensity of a noxious stimulus after applying a fake "analgesic" or "pain-enhancing" cream. In the laboratory setting, where the effects can be measured, one can expect decreases (placebo) or increases (nocebo) in pain ratings that are considered large because most of the ratings of the group "treated" with placebo or nocebo would not overlap with ratings of the untreated group.[24] Of course, the intensity of the pain-evoking stimulation used in the laboratory is far below the tissue-damaging level. Nonetheless, the neural mechanisms activated in the placebo condition are likely relevant to an understanding of the remarkably robust sports, ritual, or acupuncture analgesia discussed in Chapter 1. Likewise, the nocebo effect is obviously relevant for guiding medical practice and assessing the effectiveness of treatment.

As discussed earlier, it was known near the time of the Issaquah meeting that opiate-like (opioid) receptors were present in the CNS and that these receptors were the targets not only of opiate drugs but also of endogenous opioid compounds within the CNS. Early studies of patients undergoing dental surgery showed that naloxone, a drug that blocks the activation of opioid receptors, increases postoperative pain and attenuates the analgesic effect of a placebo, suggesting that the placebo effect is mediated by an endogenous opioid mechanism.[25] Separate follow-up studies show that nonopioid mechanisms may be involved also and that very subtle environmental cues can trigger a placebo effect that is roughly equivalent to a moderately hypalgesic effect of morphine.[26] Although these studies confirm the opioid-based pain-modulating effect of cognitive processes, a mechanistic understanding of these effects is incomplete without some understanding of the underlying neural circuitry.

Given the presence and location of opioid receptors in the brain, it was natural to investigate the possibility of a link between the structures activated during opioid-induced analgesia and the placebo effect. Early PET studies showed that opioid drugs markedly attenuate the activation of structures during pain and that some of these structures or their component parts are also active during opioid analgesia and during the placebo effect.[27] The PAG and different parts of the cingulate and prefrontal cortex, for example, are active during pain, opioid-induced analgesia, and placebo conditions. These results are consistent with an opioid-mediated analgesia mechanism that is triggered both by nociceptors in damaged tissues (a feedback control mechanism) and by cognitive processes generated in the cerebral cortex.

The PET studies were revealing, but the unique physical properties of fMRI and the BOLD response promoted the development of *connectivity analysis*, which allows investigators to go beyond simply locating multiple sites of activation and to investigate more accurately the relationships among them. Given the extensive anatomical connections and the ongoing neuronal activity within the CNS, it is important to distinguish between activations that occur together by chance and those that occur because of some causal relationship among them. As you might expect, making this distinction requires that the analysis of fMRI experiments is based on sophisticated mathematical statistics. Some types of connectivity can be interpreted simply as joint occurrences or correlations of activation without assigning a causal relationship (called "functional" connectivity), while others can be shown to have some causal relationship, indicating that activation "A," for example, significantly increases the probability of activation "B" (called "effective" connectivity). By constraining the analysis to known properties of the system (e.g., anatomical connections), it is possible to determine not only if a stimulus activates one or more CNS sites but also whether that stimulus, and perhaps the cognitive state during stimulus delivery, alters the effective connectivity among the different activations.[28] This type of analysis, called *dynamic causal modeling*, greatly enriches the investigation of functional imaging generally and of the cognitive modulation of pain in particular.

Functional MRI studies confirm the reduction of pain-related brain activations during the placebo effect and provide additional evidence, through connectivity and correlation analyses, that placebo hypalgesia is an active process that generates a top-down cascade of activations from the prefrontal cortex to the thalamus, brainstem, and spinal cord to attenuate nociceptive excitation at several levels within the CNS. It is now clear that placebo, nocebo, and other cognitive modulation effects, such as expectancy, can be mediated by, or independent of, opioid-based mechanisms and can be established by the recruitment of pathways that employ dopamine, serotonin, norepinephrine, or other molecules as neurotransmitters. Moreover, it now appears that pain facilitation or the nocebo effect is neurophysiologically distinct from the placebo mechanism and involves different forebrain and, perhaps, brainstem mechanisms.[29]

There are many other cognitive processes, such as fear, attention, expectation, and even religious belief,[30] that attenuate or facilitate the perception of pain through the activity of neural circuits that may be distinct from one another. For example, the local rCBF changes revealed by arterial spin labeling (see Chapter 9, section on "Functional Imaging: Functional Magnetic Resonance Imaging and Positron Emission Tomography") shows that the structures activated and deactivated during *mindfulness meditation hypalgesia* are different from those during placebo hypalgesia.[31] In fact, some structures may be active during either pain or hypalgesia, consistent with the limited resolution and valence ambiguity inherent in surrogate measures of neuronal activity. As suggested here, some of these modulating circuits involve endogenous opioid mechanisms, and some do not.

Connectivity analysis has begun to reveal network structures that underlie the implementation of these various cognitive effects. To summarize the complex effects of placebo, other forms of cognitive modulation, and their neurobiological foundations, I have inserted Figure 10.5,[32] which emphasizes the participation of the prefrontal cortex in the initiation of the placebo, nocebo, and other cognitive modulations.

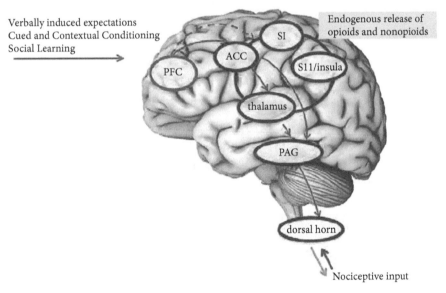

FIGURE 10.5. Summary depiction of some of the neuronal mechanisms participating in the modulation of pain during the placebo effect and other cognitive processes. A diagrammatic representation of neuronal pathways is superimposed on an image of the left cerebral hemisphere, cerebellum, brainstem, and cervical (upper or rostral) spinal cord. The major areas activated during pain are encircled in *red: ACC,* anterior cingulate cortex; *S1,* primary somatosensory cortex, *SII/insula,* secondary somatosensory cortex and insula; *PAG;* periaqueductal gray matter. Areas of the prefrontal cortex (*PFC,* encircled in *green*) are shown here as initiating attenuations of pain-related responses by direct pathways (*green solid arrows*) and by changing the connectivity among pain-activated regions (*dashed green arrow*).

From Colloca L, Klinger R, Flor H, and Bingel U. Placebo analgesia: Psychological and neurobiological mechanisms. *Pain 154*: 511–514, 2013, with permission of Wolters Kluwer Health, Inc.

PAIN OVER TIME: CHRONIC PAIN

We all learn and recall at least some of what we have learned. Obviously, the brain undergoes enduring or "plastic" physical changes at some molecular, cellular, and systems network level, or this common experience would not be possible. Although much progress has been made over the last several decades, we still have only a rudimentary grasp of the physical processes and changes that underlie the formation of everyday memories. Similarly, we have a very limited understanding of the neural mechanisms that are responsible for a different kind of plasticity: the chronic pain that persists well beyond the healing of an injury and sometimes even in the absence of an apparent injury. As noted in the Introduction, chronic pain is a major population heath problem.[33] So, why does pain sometimes persist? For that matter, why does pain usually subside? These questions are the focus of intense, ongoing investigation today.

Chronic pain is difficult to define.[34] Specifying an arbitrary time is insufficient and misleading. There are many variables that contribute to the persistence of pain, including the location and type of injury, a prolonged time of healing, ongoing inflammatory processes (in the peripheral nervous system [PNS] and CNS), the regeneration of nerve fibers in the PNS, and multiple cognitive modulations, to name just a few. In daily practice, the problem of chronic pain often comes down to choosing among pain treatments that are directed toward a presumed source of nociceptive input (the PNS) or toward modifying the perception of pain (the CNS), or that include some combination of each. Which of these choices predominates depends, of course, on the strength of evidence for a PNS source of nociceptor activity. If there is good evidence for a PNS source of ongoing nociceptive input, the therapeutic direction is clear: focus on attenuating the input by any appropriate means (e.g., anti-inflammatory measures, local or regional anesthesia) and add centrally acting analgesic medications as necessary. A problem arises when these simple measures don't work; then we may be dealing with a developing or ongoing chronic pain problem.

Common experience tells us that the intensity and quality of pain change over time even though the intensity of the stimulus remains constant. However, most functional imaging studies of pain in healthy volunteers use relatively brief noxious stimuli lasting typically less than 10 seconds; some use 2- to 20-minute periods of repetitive 5-second stimuli. Infrared laser pulses, often delivered repetitively for several seconds, last only a few milliseconds. But the pain experienced during even brief repetitive stimuli can change. For example, 3-second pulses of moderately painful heat applied to the skin are much more painful when applied every 3 seconds than every 6 seconds because there is a rapid *temporal summation* of heat nociceptor excitation of CNS neurons, a phenomenon called *windup*. As expected, imaging studies reveal greatly enhanced activations within pain-related structures during this windup.[35] A more common form of pain windup is the "hot potato" phenomenon experienced when trying to hold a hot object. Imaging studies of continuous noxious stimulation sustained for only a minute show that the spatial pattern of activation changes dramatically even though the stimulation intensity is unchanged. If moderately painful heat (48° C) is applied to the skin for 20 seconds, the sites of activation move, after about 10 seconds, from the orbitofrontal and cingulate to the insular and somatosensory cortices and the thalamus (Figure 10.6). This pattern is

Contrast effects

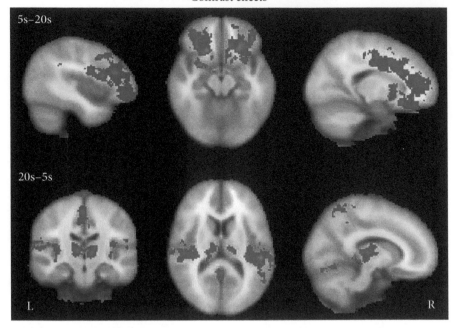

FIGURE 10.6. Changes in the spatial pattern of activations during the continuous application of moderately noxious heat (48° C) for 20 seconds. Lateral and medial hemispheres are shown on the *upper left* and *right* and on the *lower right*; a coronal section is shown on the *lower left* and *horizontal* sections in the *middle upper* and *lower panels*. *Upper* images (*left* to *right*) show lateral, orbital, and medial frontal lobe activations during the first 5 minutes in contrast to the activations after 20 seconds. *Lower* images show the thalamic and insular cortical activations after 20 seconds in contrast with the activations during the first 5 seconds.

(From Tran TD, Wang H, Tandon A, Hernandez-Garcia L, and Casey KL. Temporal summation of heat pain in humans: Evidence supporting thalamocortical modulation. *Pain 150*: 93–102, 2010, with permission of Wolters Kluwer Health, Inc.)

similar to that observed in an earlier PET study of repetitive 5-second heat pulses applied to the skin for about 100 seconds.[36] Complex temporal changes in the spatial pattern of pain-related activation are observed also during more prolonged (15–20 minutes) noxious stimuli, using acidic injections into deep tissues.[37] Thus, there is no doubt that, even in the first several seconds and minutes of exposure to a noxious stimulus, the cerebral processing of pain is a temporally and spatially dynamic process involving the active recruitment and attenuation of structures that generate and modulate the sensory, affective, and cognitive dimensions of pain. It is reasonable to expect, then, that chronic pain, which lasts much longer and has many different causes, has cerebral "signatures" that are much different from and more diverse than those identified thus far by the functional imaging of acute pain.

Among the possible CNS contributors to chronic pain is *central neuroinflammation*, which may lead to the development of *central sensitization*, as discussed in Chapter 7.[38] These processes can enhance the excitatory potential of even painless, mild, or moderate nociceptive activity so that potential PNS sources of pain may be overlooked; this is important because low-level nociceptive activity can sustain these central processes.[39] These plastic changes may take place within the cerebral network activated by acute pain. But as the foregoing functional imaging studies show, the pain-associated network may change dramatically even over seconds or minutes, creating moving targets for pain treatment. The brain is likely to undergo even more changes during chronic pain lasting days, weeks, months, or years.

The functional organization of the somatosensory cortex changes after the amputation of a limb, and this has been correlated with the phenomenon of *phantom limb pain* in the limb that is missing but persistently perceived.[40] In animal experiments, cortical neurons that previously responded only during stimulation of the preamputated limb begin to respond to stimulation of other body areas such as the face. In humans, tactile or thermal stimulation of the face evokes sensations in both the face and the phantom limb. These observations suggest that a loss of sensory input from the body leads to a facilitation or disinhibition (or both) of inputs to the affected neurons, perhaps aiding the development of chronic pain. There is now strong evidence that the pain of a phantom limb is maintained by spontaneous ongoing discharges originating in the dorsal root sensory cell bodies (ganglia) that innervated the amputated limb.[41] But why these discharges would be painful in some amputees is unknown. It is possible that central sensitization has occurred during cortical reorganization, leading to maladaptive responsiveness to ongoing, normally painless activity.[42] This conjecture is supported by evidence that cognitive processes, such as viewing a mirror image of the moving, intact limb in place of the amputated limb, reduces phantom limb pain and alters cortical responsiveness.[43]

In other chronic pain conditions, the spatial pattern of brain activation and the distribution of response intensity show distinct differences from those observed during experimentally induced pain in healthy individuals. "Low back pain" (LBP) is among the most common chronic pain problems.[44] On a population level, LBP is caused by a mixture of nociceptive inputs from injured muscle, skeletal, joint, and connective tissues; sometimes there is evidence for nerve injury also. Functional MRI studies of patients with LBP for a year or more[45] show that, during exacerbations of their back pain, the predominant brain activations are in the medial prefrontal cortex and in limbic system-related structures that, collectively, are associated with the cognitive and affective dimensions of the pain experience. Similar results are observed in other conditions such as the chronic pain that sometimes follows herpetic neuralgia ("shingles"). The exact pattern of brain activation varies according to the clinical condition; some of the responses are either outside the acute pain network or are amplified activations within it. In any event, it appears that the brain during chronic pain is different from the healthy brain during acute pain. The difference, moreover, is not restricted to responses evoked by pain because there is evidence that the default or resting state of the brain is different during chronic pain. An fMRI study of LBP patients showed that they *deactivate* the medial prefrontal cortex less than normal individuals during a cognitive task and also exhibit reduced functional connectivity of these sites with other cortical areas.[46] This does not mean that the brain changes observed in chronic pain necessarily cause the pain to persist or that the changes are indelible; it strongly suggests, however, that the treatment of chronic pain is more likely to be effective if it takes into account these brain response differences and the patient's experience that accompanies them.

Pain causes, and is affected by, structural changes in the brain. Voxel-based morphometry (VBM; see Chapter 9, section on "Some Essential Background") is used to estimate the amount of gray matter (neurons and glial cells vs. white matter and fluid) in the brain. In normal, healthy individuals, these gray matter estimates appear to have a complex relationship with measures of pain sensitivity. Depending on how pain sensitivity is measured (pain threshold vs. suprathreshold pain rating), some brain regions show either a positive or negative correlation of pain sensitivity with the thickness or density of gray matter.[47] Also, repetitive painful heat stimulation, delivered for 20 minutes daily to normal individuals for 8 consecutive days, increases heat pain threshold, reduces the rating of pain intensity, and increases gray matter for about 3 weeks before returning to normal within a year.[48] These findings suggest that, whatever their physiological basis, pain-induced gray matter changes may be temporary. Nonetheless, VBM studies generally reveal long-term (years) reductions of gray matter, primarily in the prefrontal or frontal lobe cortex, among groups of patients with various types of chronic pain (Figure 10.7).[49]

These gray matter losses are accompanied by biochemical changes that are consistent with a loss of neuronal and/or glial cells. In a clinically well-defined group of patients with chronic pain following nerve damage, the gray matter loss is at least partially attributable to a loss of small interneurons containing the inhibitory neurotransmitter gamma-aminobutyric acid (GABA) There is evidence suggesting that, in some forms of

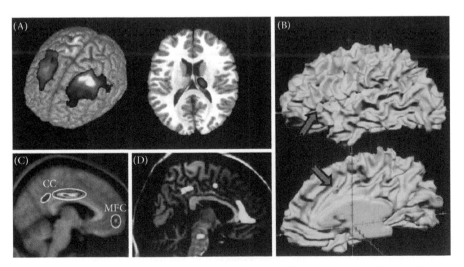

FIGURE 10.7. Localized decreases in gray matter as determined by voxel-based morphometry in clinical chronic pain conditions. (A) Chronic back pain (bilateral dorsolateral prefrontal cortex and thalamus). (B) Irritable bowel syndrome (insular cortex, *upper arrow*; cingulate cortex, *lower arrow*). (C) Fibromyalgia (cingulate cortex and medial prefrontal cortex). (D) Chronic tension headache (multifocal cingulate cortex and upper brainstem).

From Apkarian AV, Hashmi JA, and Baliki MN. Pain and the brain: Specificity and plasticity of the brain in clinical chronic pain. *Pain 152:* S49–S64, 2011, with permission of Wolters Kluwer Health, Inc.

chronic pain associated with nerve damage, a loss of normal inhibitory control leads to the development of abnormal oscillatory connectivity within somatosensory and limbic system structures.[50] Whether this specific pathophysiology applies to many other cases of chronic pain is at best uncertain; and a fully unifying picture of the issue seems unlikely at present, in part because it is difficult to establish a firm causal relationship between chronic pain and changes in gray matter volume.[51]

For now, it is perhaps best to acknowledge that prolonged nociceptive input is associated with a pattern of brain activation that is often different from that observed during acute pain and can change brain structure and connectivity, at least temporarily, and that these responses of the CNS should be considered in planning and researching the treatment of chronic pain. It is not possible currently to use anatomical or functional brain imaging as a substitute indicator or surrogate measure of the patient's report of either acute or chronic pain.[52]

FUNCTIONAL BRAIN IMAGING: A SUMMARIZING COMMENT

Images of the living human brain have revolutionized neuroscience and medicine. Anatomical imaging allows a direct comparison of clinical conditions with the location of focal or distributed destructive brain lesions. These observations confirm earlier studies showing that pain does not have a single, unique CNS location but is instead distributed among several sites with functions other than, or in addition to, the creation of pain. Functional imaging with PET and fMRI enriches this information. We can now locate an assembly of CNS structures that become active and interactive in complex ways during pain. We can measure this activity and its connectivity and show how emotional and cognitive processes contribute to and modify pain and the responses of the multiple neural structures that somehow create it. We see evidence that brain structure and pain interact in complex ways that are likely to be very important for understanding a major clinical problem: chronic pain. We seem to be coming close to capturing pain and ending the chase that began centuries ago, was organized in a remote setting near Issaquah over 40 years ago, and continues even more intensely to the present. So why does the chase continue?

11

UNFINISHED BUSINESS

A SAMPLE

The more we chase, the more we realize that we have not captured pain in a way that fully satisfies the medical, neuroscientific, or philosophical goals suggested at the beginning of Chapter 2. Yet, we have come a long way since the Issaquah meeting. We should no longer have an oversimplified conceptual model that misdirects medical practice and scientific inquiry. Still, we do not yet have the ideal analgesic agent, one that would provide complete pain relief without addiction or other unwanted side effects, that has a controlled site and duration of action, and that is safe, inexpensive, and easy to administer. Furthermore, faulty conceptual models still lead to misguided, ineffective interventions and medical errors. Of particular concern is the recent rise in the United States and elsewhere of opioid abuse and of deaths from prescription opioid overdose.[1] And we are far from being able to specify the exact anatomical and chemical brain condition that causes pain as a subset of conscious experiences; and we are even farther from fully understanding, at a physical level, how brains, and specifically human brains, perform all the functions that can be identified—from relatively simple reflexive behaviors to complex cognitive tasks.

At least part of the problem may be technical. After all, the development of the sophisticated techniques discussed thus far has taken us in a fruitful direction. Maybe more refined and detailed imaging combined with biochemical analysis and more sophisticated psychophysical measurements will provide unexpected insights. Perhaps technical advances we cannot yet imagine will allow us to achieve the goals suggested here and even beyond.

But maybe not. Here are a few, but only a few, items of unfinished business (in no particular order).

HEADACHE

In common usage, the word "headache" refers to a deep, aching, sometimes throbbing, and often poorly localized head pain lasting more than several hours. In their 2013 International Classification of Headache Disorders,[2] the International Headache Society lists 64 types of *primary* headaches, namely, those that do not have an obvious cause such as trauma or infection (those that do are called *secondary* headaches). The most common types of primary headache are migraine (about 23 types) and "tension-type" headache (about 9 types). Most people reading this book will have had one or more of these headaches at some time in their lives. Given the intimidating taxonomy of headaches, I will severely restrict my comments to limited aspects of the most common ones.

Migraine headache is one manifestation of the migraine *syndrome*, which consists, in a common form, of a headache that is often poorly localized to one side of the head, perhaps around an eye, and sometimes accompanied by tearing or facial flushing. The headache is often preceded or accompanied by a variety of symptoms, called an *aura*, which may include mood changes, sensitivity to light or sound, flickering visual images, other sensory experiences, and nausea or vomiting.[3] Patients may have only one or a few of these symptoms, some may have none, and a few may have some of these symptoms but without headache. The variable association of auras with headache is evidence that the aura experience is neither necessary nor sufficient for generating the headache. However, the existence of these auras suggests a disturbance that is widely distributed within the brain. This conjecture is supported by the occurrence of widespread *allodynia* during a migraine attack; the scalp, facial skin, and even remote parts of the body may feel unpleasant and almost painful to touch.[4]

Tension-type headache is often characterized as a band-like pressure around the entire head.[5] Unlike migraine headache, it is not preceded by sensory or mood-related aura and usually not accompanied by other sensory symptoms or autonomic disturbances. The headache may be periodic and of variable frequency or, in the worst cases, may occur every day for long periods. Chronic daily headache, when severe, is often associated with depression and other psychological disturbances, but it is difficult to establish a clear cause-and-effect relationship.

We remain uncertain about the tissue source for the pain in these most common headaches. For many years, the prevailing view was that migraine headache was caused by the distention of cranial blood vessel walls, which are known to possess nociceptors and to evoke pain when stimulated. It was thought that effective treatments were those that constricted these dilated vessels. The pulsating, throbbing pain experienced during many migraine headaches was attributed to the repetitive stretch of dilated blood vessels. Some imaging studies reveal a correlation between these vascular changes, migraine headache, and responses to treatment, but like most correlation studies, it is not possible to establish a clear cause-and-effect relationship. Recent vascular imaging studies show that the dilation and constriction of cranial blood vessels is not related to migraine headache pain (or its relief) and that the sensation of throbbing does not coincide with the pulsation of blood vessels.[6] Furthermore, the most effective drugs for treating migraine headache, the calcitonin gene–related peptide (CGRP) receptor antagonists and serotonin receptor agonists (triptans), are not analgesic for other painful conditions and appear to relieve migraine (but not tension-type) headache by central nervous system (CNS) mechanisms unrelated to the constriction of blood vessels.[7] Another possible source for the pain of migraine headache is the sensory fibers of the meninges covering the brain. The occasional therapeutic effect of cranial botulinum toxin injections partially supports this hypothesis because the toxin reduces the release of sensory neurotransmitters, a mechanism similar to that of the triptans.[8] Still, we remain uncertain about the source of migraine headache pain. Moreover, whatever the origin of the sensory inputs creating the pain of migraine, we do not understand why or how these inputs should periodically become painful. One current hypothesis, which recalls the preceding discussion of central sensitization (see Chapter 7), is that the migraine syndrome reflects a wide-spread enhancement of neuronal sensitivity within central sensory pathways caused by an episodic dysfunction of brainstem modulatory mechanisms, possibly mediated by CNS peptides such as CGRP (see earlier). This hypothesis is challenged, however, by evidence that the clinically effective triptan compounds are poor penetrators of the blood-brain barrier (see the Appendix), suggesting a peripheral site of their therapeutic action.[9] Furthermore, the proximal cause of these proposed hypersensitivity episodes remains unknown. Nonetheless, the overall clinical evidence seems to favor an increase in neuronal activity in CNS somatic and visceral sensory circuits, perhaps by a temporary loss of neuronal inhibitory control, causing pain.

In the case of tension-type headache, the story is similar, but the pathophysiology is even more obscure. The putative cause, "tension," is thought by some to be a combination of psychological stress and chronic constriction of muscles around the face and scalp. Although some studies show a correlation between the pain of "tension" headache and various psychophysiological measurements, such as scalp muscle tenderness, it is not possible to determine why these muscles should become tender; perhaps central sensitization is involved here also, but its cause is also unknown.[10] There is speculation that tension-type and migraine headache have similar physiological pathologies in part because, in some patients, episodic migraine can be "transformed" into a chronic headache condition that is clinically similar to tension-type headache.

In summary, because a source of painful nociceptor input from the skin, blood vessels, or muscles of the head is not yet established for these headaches, it appears that, in both migraine and tension-type headache, some part of the pain-generating circuitry in the CNS may become abnormally active and excitable. How and why this abnormal activity develops remain to be determined. Identifying the neural circuitry that generates these common headaches would be a major advance in the chase for pain.

THE LIMBIC SYSTEM REVISITED: A CASE REPORT

It is rare that the careful study of a single patient changes or significantly affects the direction of an entire field of inquiry. The study of the late patient Henry Molaison (1926–2008) is an example of how investigating the neurobiology of memory was greatly influenced by the careful analysis of the effect of a focal lesion in the human brain.[11] Although there are other clinical cases that have had an impact on thinking about pain (see Chapter 3), a patient recently described in great detail may force the medical and neuroscientific communities to revisit current conceptual models of pain mechanisms generally and of the contribution of the limbic system particularly (at least as originally defined and currently conceived). The case report summarized below represents a fortunate confluence of detailed observational narrative and anatomical brain imaging; its impact derives from the frequency with which the cingulate and insular cortices are identified by some as critical, even essential, for the experience of pain.[12]

In 1975, a 48-year-old man ("patient B") developed severe herpes simplex encephalitis.[13] This form of encephalitis commonly damages the brain's temporal lobe and the associated limbic cortex. Detailed analysis of anatomical magnetic resonance imaging (MRI) brain studies (obtained during the observation period long after the acute infection) revealed severe damage of both insular cortices (described as "entirely destroyed") and most of the cingulate, orbitofrontal, hippocampal, and adjacent temporal lobe cortices of both hemispheres; the amygdalae (gray matter structures at the tips of the temporal lobes) were also destroyed. The parietal and somatosensory cortices (S1 and S2), thalamus, subcortical basal ganglia (in front of the thalamus; see the Appendix), hypothalamus, and upper brainstem were largely or completely spared. His most obvious neurologic deficit was a severe loss of recent (episodic) memory. Although detailed psychophysical tests of pain and somesthetic function are not presented in this report, the patient's clinical sensory examination was normal, and he readily complained of pain and expressed a fear of pain associated with needle injections, removal of adhesive tape, and other common encounters with noxious stimuli. He responded normally to tickling. Extensive testing and daily observation of his behavior revealed complete self-awareness and a full range of affective experiences from anger and sadness to joy.

This patient felt and feared pain without most of his limbic cortex. The insular, cingulate, and orbitofrontal cortices of both hemispheres were either completely destroyed or extensively damaged. His full range of affective feelings and of painful experiences depended instead on intact frontal, parietal, and somatosensory cortices acting together with subcortical limbic structures such as the hypothalamus, parts of the basal ganglia, and neural structures in the upper brainstem, including the periaqueductal gray and adjacent reticular formation. The authors of this article acknowledge that, except for the presumed retrograde degeneration of thalamocortical projection neurons, this patient's thalamus was intact; however, they discounted its potential role in pain and affect by suggesting that it serves only as an "information conduit from brainstem" (p. 11) to the brain. Perhaps, as these authors suggest, the cortical structures missing in this patient serve primarily to provide more abstract cognitive elaborations of affective experience such as imagination or the recognition of emotion (and pain) in others.[14] Perhaps intact basal ganglia structures such as the nucleus accumbens and its subcortical connections are sufficient to provide at least some affective component of a range of experiences including pain.[15]

It is extremely rare to have extensive bilateral insular damage while retaining the ability to participate in extensive cognitive and neurological evaluations as described earlier; indeed, only two such cases have been extensively tested and reported in the literature. In the additional patient (male patient "R"),[16] the insular and anterior cingulate cortical damage was complete on the right and 78% and 99% damaged, respectively, on the left. There was also extensive damage of the midline (medial) prefrontal cortex. Functional connectivity of the medial prefrontal and remaining left insular cortex was absent. This patient had severe deficits in memory, olfaction, and taste consistent with damage to the hippocampus, the "taste cortex" part of the insula, and related limbic structures. Extensive testing of somatosensory function revealed no deficits. However, this patient, compared with control subjects, was unable to detect a change in his heart rate after local anesthesia of his chest skin, and he had less robust ratings of the affective impact of a set of emotion-evoking images. These latter results suggest that the insular cortex participates in visceral sensory mechanisms and in modulating the level of an existing emotional awareness.

An earlier psychophysical and functional MRI (fMRI) study of two patients with unilateral (left side) insular stroke damage confirms the observation that an intact insular cortex is not necessary for the perception of pain.[17] Indeed, these patients were able to discriminate among different intensities of heat applied to either side of the body and had *increased* ratings of painful heat applied to the affected (right) side. Functional imaging revealed *increased* activation intensities of the somatosensory cortex compared with normal subjects.

The insular cortex has received a great deal of attention in recent years, due largely to the heuristic hypothesis that it functions as an "interoceptive cortex," receiving and integrating a wide range of visceral and somatic information to provide our sense of self-awareness.[18] Some aspects of patient R's examination and recent functional imaging studies support this conjecture. And partial functionality, whatever that might mean for self-experience and behavior, could possibly be retained by small amounts of spared insular tissue. However, based on the previous case reports, the wide variety of sensory inputs to the insula, and the multiple diverse clinical effects of insular lesions, it appears that this cortical structure may be best regarded as modulating emotional responses to internal and external sensory inputs. Normal insular function is not necessary for pain nor for the degree of self-awareness consistent with daily living.

Whatever other interpretations might be applied to these particular case reports, it seems that a fully intact limbic cortical circuitry is not necessary for physical pain as we humans normally experience it. Most of the frontal lobe cortex and all of the parietal and occipital cortex remained intact in these patients and could participate, along with the remaining thalamic, basal ganglia, and upper brainstem structures, in the generation of their apparently normal pain experiences. The conjoint activity of the somatosensory (S1 and S2) cortex and subcortical structures with a close functional connection to the hypothalamus may also be necessary for pain, but this cannot be determined unequivocally with the data at hand. Some small portion of the cingulate cortex may have been incompletely damaged in these patients and could still be functioning.[19] However, the extensive emotional circuitry defined by Papez and MacLean[20] appears to be more elaborate than necessary for physical pain. The hypothalamic, upper brainstem circuitry of Philip Bard's "sham rage" cats[21] is certainly too sparse. Pain is presumably somewhere in between. More elaborate and detailed functional imaging alone is unlikely to give the answer. So, the chase for pain continues.

ANESTHESIA AWARENESS

Imagine you are undergoing abdominal surgery. The anesthesiologist has administered an intravenous drug that has presumably rendered you unconscious; this has been supplemented with an inhaled anesthetic gas administered first through a face mask and later by a tube inserted down your trachea. You are intravenously administered an agent that blocks the chemical (acetylcholine) connection between your motor nerves and skeletal muscles (neuromuscular blockade), thus paralyzing you completely. As the surgery begins, you become aware of snippets of conversation around the operating table. Soon, you experience the sudden, sharp, excruciating pain of the scalpel progressing down your belly, followed by a deeper, tearing pain as the subcutaneous tissue is removed to expose abdominal muscles. You want desperately to scream, to stop this torture, but you are helpless, immobilized, and unable to communicate in any way as the surgery proceeds as though nothing is wrong. Then there is the unbearable deep cramping pain as the abdominal muscles are stretched, followed by diffuse, nauseating cramping, more intense than any "gas pains" you have ever experienced, as your intestines are manipulated. This goes on unabated for an hour or more, ending only after you experience repeated piercing and stretching as your skin is sown together when the abdominal wound is closed.

Horrible experiences like this occur very rarely but they do occur, more commonly consisting of shorter, incomplete stretches of awareness. According to a review of incidence,[22] anesthesia awareness with recall (AWR) occurs during one or two of 1000 surgeries performed under general anesthesia. The experience of pain is recalled, within one to two weeks after surgery, by nearly 30% of those with AWR. The authors estimate that, given the number of surgeries requiring general anesthesia, 26,000 patients will experience AWR each year in the United States. That incidence means that approximately 100 AWR events, with three experiencing pan, will occur each workday. This problem would go unnoticed, of course, if the individuals who have experienced it did not remember it and had not reported it to their doctors. (Or lawyers!) It is nonetheless a nightmare for those few who have had such experiences and a possibility, however remote, deeply feared by those who have heard about "awake anesthesia" and are about to undergo surgery themselves. Anesthesiologists are likewise deeply concerned about this problem and are continuing to conduct research into the cause (or causes) of the problem. Unfortunately, although progress has been made, we still do not understand the neural mechanisms that allow people who appear completely unconscious to experience pain.

Can AWR be avoided? Currently, there are no reliable criteria for predicting whether a patient will or will not experience AWR. An American Society of Anesthesiologists Task Force lists some risk factors such as a history of AWR, a history of substance abuse, and various physiological conditions associated with chronic vascular or pulmonary diseases, but the presence or absence of any one of these does not reliably predict the occurrence of AWR.[23]

Can AWR be stopped? Detecting the presence of AWR is very difficult. Postoperative interviews require answers to specific questions asked in the recovery suite as well as a week or more thereafter to assure the reliability of the responses and to differentiate dreaming from the recollection of specific intraoperative events.[24] But detecting AWR after the fact does little to solve the problem. Monitoring the electroencephalogram (EEG) would seem to be a rational choice for detecting AWR during surgery, but this is not fully reliable in part because drug effects and uncontrolled physiological variables can cloud the interpretation of changes in the EEG.[25]

Because of evidence that the shift between conscious and unconscious states can be detected by monitoring changes in the temporal coherence among different rhythmic EEG waveforms, a bispectral index scale (BIS) has become available for use with a proprietary monitoring device. The BIS provides a single number as an indicator of consciousness and is currently employed during surgeries at several institutions throughout the world. Although the BIS is reported to be useful in several surgical settings, a recent review indicates that even this method lacks sufficient reliability to recommend its use as the only monitor for anesthesia awareness.[26] Accordingly, to reduce the incidence of AWR, it is common practice to maintain a minimum alveolar concentration (MAC) of volatile anesthetic gas sufficient to suppress reflexive withdrawal from a noxious stimulus in a nonparalyzed patient.

The problem of AWR makes it a practical necessity to achieve the best possible understanding of the neural mechanisms of anesthesia, consciousness, and pain. To begin, it is necessary to realize that the pharmacologically induced surgical anesthetic state is quite different from natural sleep and is likely to be different from any of several other states of unconsciousness induced by various agents or methods such as trauma, asphyxia, low blood glucose, and carbon monoxide. The neural circuits that are targeted by various anesthetic agents are different from one another and markedly different from those affected during conscious analgesia. As noted previously and indicated by AWR itself, anesthesia does not guarantee analgesia and analgesia certainly does not require anesthesia.

Anesthetic agents administered intravenously or by inhalation act at different and multiple sites. Some agents are known to enhance the effects of the inhibitory neurotransmitter gamma-aminobutyric acid (GABA), while others primarily reduce the excitatory effects of glutamate or acetylcholine on their respective neuronal receptors. Through their action on a widely distributed group of G protein–coupled neuronal membrane receptors, different anesthetic agents can also affect the action of other neurotransmitters such as dopamine, serotonin, and norepinephrine. Given the widespread and varying distribution of these neurotransmitter systems in the CNS, it appears that anesthetic agents do not have a single or highly restricted mode of action at the molecular level.[27]

Perhaps a common mode of anesthetic action can be detected at the systems or circuit level. This possibility returns us again to the EEG, which has the strong practical advantage of being recordable from scalp electrodes during a surgical procedure. Since the turn of the millennium, there has been a strong interest in rhythmic EEG activity within the range of 30 to 90 Hz, commonly called the *gamma frequency* or *gamma band*. These rhythmic microvolt amplitude waves, as recorded from scalp electrodes, are found in several regions of the cerebral cortex, including the S1 and S2 somatosensory cortices and are thought to be generated by the summed, synchronous synaptic activity of cortical neurons interacting with neurons in the thalamus and other cortical areas. Thus, the presence of gamma band activity is widely regarded as evidence for the active formation of the connectivity necessary for integrated sensory, motor, and cognitive functions. Recent evidence from EEG, magnetoencephalogram (MEG), and laser evoked potential (LEP) recordings indicates that gamma activity in the S1 somatosensory cortex, for example, is preferentially evoked by noxious laser heat stimulation that correlates strongly with perceived pain intensity.[28] Overall, the evidence indicates that pain requires the conjoint activity of widely distributed groups of neurons; it also suggests the possibility that gamma activity or some related measure could be used to detect the cerebral conditions necessary and sufficient for AWR and for the perception of pain specifically. However, many practical and technical issues must be addressed before the clinical practicality of gamma band monitoring can be tested adequately.[29]

PAIN, CONSCIOUSNESS, AND SUFFERING AT
THE BEDSIDE

Between 10,000 and 40,000 individuals in the United States are currently estimated to be in a vegetative state (VS; aka: unresponsive wakefulness syndrome, or UWS) because of severe brain damage from one or more among multiple causes such as trauma, stroke, drug overdose, or incomplete cardiac resuscitation.[30] Unlike patients who are paralyzed but able to communicate with eye movements or facial expressions, all VS patients are unable to communicate any inner experiences they may have. Yet VS patients typically cycle through what appear to be stages of sleep and wakefulness with their eyes open and moving. They occasionally move their limbs, grasp or push away objects, and make various facial expressions and wordless vocalizations without apparent purpose or relation to surrounding events. Patients in a related but less severe minimally conscious state (MCS) occasionally show evidence of some environmental awareness for brief periods. The number of patients in MCS cannot be estimated because of inadequate reporting and diagnostic uncertainty.

In this unfortunate setting, the patient's friends and family members often ask physicians, nurses, and other health care professionals (1) whether the patient will recover and (2) if the patient can experience pain or (3) is suffering. Neurologists, neurosurgeons, and others with neurological training are sometimes called by other professionals to counsel on this issue. Occasionally, it becomes a serious legal and even political issue.[31] Fortunately, there is evidence that the results of a standardized bedside examination may assist in answering the first two questions. By recording and scaling the patient's responses to a quantifiable, harmless noxious stimulus, trained professionals can distinguish patients in a constant VS from those with evidence of intermittent environmental awareness (MCS); this could lead to prognostic estimates that may be more reliable than those currently employed.[32] An answer to the second and third questions, however, is impossible because it requires an understanding of the neurobiology of consciousness, a necessary condition for pain or suffering. My own approach is to take an agnostic position on the second question but assure the questioners that the caregiving team will do everything possible to avoid and treat conditions that could reasonably be assumed to be painful.[33] Unfortunately, this approach does not address the more difficult third question of whether the patient may be constantly or frequently in a state similar to what we call suffering (with or without pain). We may never be able to answer this third question, but attempts to find an answer may provide some insight into the neurobiology of consciousness and, therefore, pain and perhaps AWR.

CONSCIOUSNESS AND THE CONCEPTUAL
MODEL REVISITED

The experiments of Sherrington and Bard (see Chapter 4) showed that, in cats and dogs, "pseudaffective" defensive behaviors and even spontaneous directed attacks require only an intact brainstem, thalamus, and hypothalamus. Although these animals did not continually engage in proactive (anticipatory) exploration and were generally quiet between evoking stimuli, they were not entirely stimulus-bound and occasionally made aggressive movements. These early studies implicate the upper brainstem and its immediate subcortical connections as *structures critical for supporting spontaneous interactions with the environment,* a condition that I will call "preliminary consciousness." Preliminary consciousness, as I use this term here, refers to a state of the CNS during which spontaneous, apparently purposeless movements produce pseudaffective interactions with noxious features of the environment without evincing accompanying or delayed behaviors (such as learned avoidance and spontaneous directed attacks) that suggest an experience of pain; it is at the lower end of poorly demarcated *levels of* consciousness.[34]

To make explicit the concept of levels of consciousness and the structural, behavioral, and experiential features that accompany them, I have inserted Table 11.1. The grayed row in this table reflects the gray area of our understanding of the transition from the unconscious to the fully conscious state. As I have defined preliminary consciousness here, the structures do not include the cerebral cortex.

In this table, connectivity refers to both functional and effective connectivity (see Chapter 10) among subcortical and cortical structures, possibly detected as gamma frequency oscillations. The term "pseudoexploratory" is intended to convey the idea of random or apparently purposeless, contacts with the environment, driven by the *intrinsic property of movement generation in animals.* In this view, active subcortical structures in the upper brainstem, thalamus, basal ganglia, and hypothalamus initiate movements that contact the environment, stimulating sensory receptors (including nociceptors), thus initiating both reflexive feedback control and the subsequent *recruitment of cortical structures* for anticipatory or *proactive* guidance of exploration. At the transitional level from preliminary to full consciousness, the degree and content of inner experience, if any, would be severely limited and beyond our capacity to imagine.[35]

Studies of VS and MCS patients reveal the primary role of subcortical structures in maintaining a condition of apparent wakefulness without evidence for environmental awareness.[36] The structural and functional CNS damage in VS patients has been investigated extensively by electrophysiological and brain imaging methods and rarely by autopsy examination of the brain.[37] The results of these studies reveal extensive cortical and subcortical damage that varies considerably depending on the cause of the brain injury (e.g., loss of blood flow, trauma, or metabolic disturbances). Therefore, this type of information alone cannot identify the structures that are most critical for preliminary consciousness. However, these investigations commonly highlight the importance of an

Table 11.1. Levels of Consciousness and Their Neurophysiological, Behavioral, and Experiential Associations

CONSCIOUSNESS	STRUCTURES	CONNECTIVITY	BEHAVIOR	EXPERIENCE
None	Spinal	Minimal	Reflexive	None
Preliminary	+ Subcortical	Limited	Pseudoexploratory	Limited
Full	+ Cortical	Full	Proactive	Full

See also: Akerman et al (2011) op. cit.

See also: Denton (2005) op. cit.

intact group of *upper brainstem, hypothalamic, thalamic, basal ganglia, cortical cingulate, parietal, and frontal lobe* structures for maintaining a state of personal and environmental awareness above that seen in the behavior of VS patients. The *subcortical* structures, because of their widespread reciprocal physiological interactions with the cerebral cortex, have global behavioral effects that are critical for consciousness. It is the *conjoint* activity within the group of subcortical structures that appears to establish the core features of the preliminary conscious state from which full consciousness develops. Given this background, the findings of a recent positron emission tomography (PET) study (discussed later) are of considerable interest.

Healthy human volunteers gradually recovered from unconsciousness induced in different experiments by two different intravenous anesthetics. Each volunteer kept his or her eyes closed unless otherwise requested. The emergence of consciousness was defined as the ability to open the eyes on command. The results showed that the return of consciousness coincides with neuronal activity in the *upper brainstem, hypothalamus, thalamus, and anterior cingulate cortex*. In addition, *connectivity* between the *parietal cortex, basal forebrain (ganglia), cingulate, and frontal lobe cortex* is established as consciousness reappears. The relevant images are shown in Figure 11.1.[38] The capacity to experience pain was not examined in these studies. The participating subjects recognized and responded to a verbal command by opening their eyes. Therefore, it is reasonable to assume that they would be capable of experiencing pain.

A related fMRI study of levels of consciousness among brain-damaged patients, including those in VS, confirms these observations by revealing the primary importance of "salience network" components, but also including insular and posterior cingulate cortex connectivity, in establishing a fully conscious state. Functional brain imaging studies have revealed some preserved but impaired effective connectivity and some cortical activations driven by verbal command in a few patients. but the degree to which these remnants of function could maintain an inner experience is at best uncertain.[39] Overall, the imaging studies support the conjecture that activity within the upper brainstem and functionally connected subcortical structures mediates preliminary consciousness and is essential for establishing the additional cortical activity that supports full consciousness. Additional support comes from a study of patients with coma caused by an upper brainstem lesion at a site that is functionally connected with the insular and cingulate cortices.[40] It is notable that this group of structures includes elements of the salience network activated during pain, and it is on this foundation that the neuronal apparatus for pain is constructed.

The evidence from these and other sources discussed previously begins to outline a subcortical-cortical circuit that provides the substrate for pseudoexploratory interactions with the environment, a feature of preliminary consciousness as I have defined it and a foundation for the capacity to experience pain. Whether this information will ultimately prove helpful in avoiding or detecting AWR, or in assisting in the care of VS and MCS patients, remains to be determined.

Full consciousness with "awareness," a term often used for the highest level of consciousness with a vivid recognition of self, extrapersonal detail, and pain, appears to

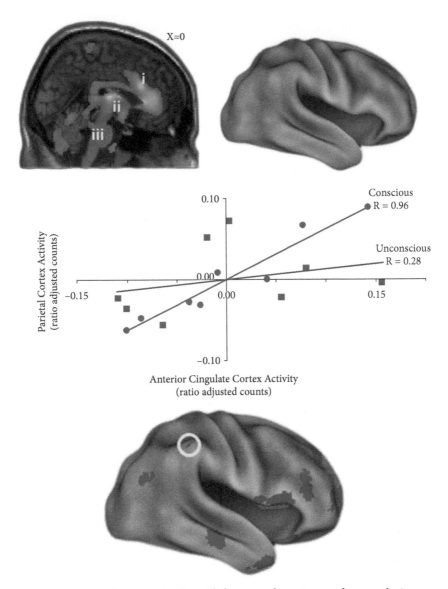

FIGURE 11.1. Neuronal activity coincident with the return of consciousness from anesthesia induced by two different intravenous agents. *Top left*: Inner (medial) surface of the left hemisphere viewed from the midline (x = 0), showing the highest levels of activation (*yellow > orange*) in the anterior cingulate cortex (i), thalamus and hypothalamus (ii), and upper brainstem (iii). *Top right*: Absence of comparable activity in other cortical structures. *Middle* and *lower*: Graph shows greater functional connectivity between the anterior cingulate cortex and the parietal cortex (*yellow circle* in *lower* image) during consciousness. Ordinate and abscissa axes show the ratios of activation intensity; R is the correlation coefficient.

Adapted from Långsjö JW, Alkire MT, Kaskinoro KD, Hayama H, Maksimow A, Kaisti KK, Aalto S, Aantaa R, Jääskeläinen SK, Revonsuo A, and Scheinin H. Returning from oblivion: Imaging the neural core of consciousness. *Journal of Neuroscience 32*: 4935–4943, 2012, with permission of the Society for Neuroscience).

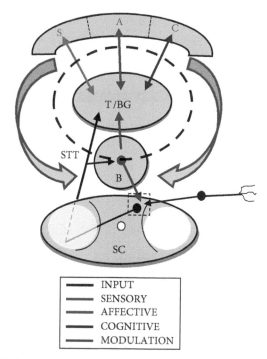

FIGURE 11.2. The *dashed circle* includes structures supporting preliminary consciousness as defined in the text: thalamus (T), basal ganglia (BG), upper brainstem (B), and hypothalamus (not shown). The basal ganglia have been added here because of the foregoing evidence for the participation of these subcortical gray matter structures in generating an affective component of experience. Modified from Figure 8.

emerge with the activation of cortical structures that process additional specific sensory and motor information. As noted previously, the activation of sensory, affective, and cognitive components of pain occurs largely in parallel and is spatially distributed.[41]

The question of the degree and quality of inner experience that may accompany subcortically mediated preliminary consciousness remains open. We may never have the tools (including brains) to answer the question (aka: the "hard problem") of how subjectivity (inner experience) arises from the activity of neurons—whatever their number and however simple or complex their organization may be.[42]

To include the importance of consciousness in a conceptual model of pain, I have made a simple addition to the model diagram of Figure 5.2 (see Chapter 5). As shown in Figure 11.2, the presence of consciousness is represented by the *dashed oval* encircling the subcortical structures mediating both preliminary consciousness and the activation of the salience-pain network. The intent here is to indicate simply that activity in the *encircled* structures includes the emergence or presence of preliminary consciousness, a necessary condition for the emergence of full consciousness and pain. As discussed previously, the close physiological and experiential connection between consciousness and pain becomes an important issue in some clinically relevant circumstances.

12

THE CHASE TODAY
SUMMARY AND IMPLICATIONS

A BRIEF RECAPITULATION

Over the more than 40 years since a chase began by organizing a group of researchers near Issaquah, Washington, we have seen the conceptual model of pain change dramatically with the development of new investigative tools and the presentation of new hypotheses to be tested. Before the Issaquah meeting, the concept of pain as a separate group of neurons with a private pathway and a localized center in the brain had been challenged, although not erased, by clinical evidence and the results of experiments on animals. Still, the conceptual simplicity and practical promise of this concept made it attractive and persistent. The alternative concept seemed to be shrouded in vague speculations about patterns and ill-defined circuitry. The gap between these ideas approached a chasm, and a bridge was difficult to imagine.

Based on the concept of functional localization as applied to pain, parts of the central nervous system (CNS) and peripheral nervous system (PNS) were destroyed for pain relief. The results showed that pain was not completely relieved, that pain or other unpleasant sensations reappeared, that other neurological functions were impaired, and that pain was also affected by lesions placed outside of putative, "classical" pain pathways. The idea that pain emerged instead through the participation of multiple CNS structures and pathways began to receive some attention.

Some relief from pain had been found to follow the consumption of extracts of plants such as the poppy, the bark of willow trees, the coca plant, hemp, and many others. Although hypalgesia could be achieved to some degree, these compounds collectively also produced a variety of side effects that included euphoria or other changes in mood, addiction, somnolence, suppression of respiration, cognitive impairment, and impaired intestinal function. Attempts to find or produce analgesic compounds without side effects failed. The existence of side effects suggested that the chemical mediators of pain relief, and therefore of pain itself, may be acting on structures distributed widely within as well as outside the CNS.

The observation that distraction, reassurance, and religious or ritualistic practices could relieve pain has a long, even ancient, history. Often, these interventions include the insertion of needles, the application of hot cups, and poultices placed on the body (see Chapter 1). For most of recorded history, the application of these methods for pain relief was either purely empirical or based on spiritual theories or their equivalents. With the early dawn of what is now called neuroscience, it became possible to consider that a substantial part of the hypalgesic effect of these practices could originate within the nervous system.

At the time of the Issaquah meeting more than 40 years ago, the ghosts of some of the foregoing ideas were present. Attempts to physically destroy pain centers or pathways had many sincere and active advocates but also many doubters. The era of molecular pharmacology was in its early phase, buoyed by the hope that just the right molecule with just the right shape would find its way to a unique receptor in the CNS or PNS and eliminate pain and pain alone with exquisite specificity and selectivity. This goal continues to elude us, but the underlying concept persists today. The idea of using the nervous system's endogenous physiological properties to attenuate pain was nascent, hidden in the shadow of more easily conceived physical and chemical interventions that were being practiced or developed.

The discovery of nociceptors in the PNS reinforced the concept of a private pain pathway and mechanism. The presence of high-threshold, inflammation-sensitive PNS receptors and nerve fibers in the skin and deep tissues is obviously important for detecting impending or actual tissue damage, so it is natural to assume that this property is sufficient for pain and that this information in the PNS is preserved "as is" in the CNS (the "labeled line"). However, the concept of specific coding by nociceptors runs into the complication of "polymodal" responses of many, perhaps most, single nociceptive fibers to various combinations of thermal, mechanical, and chemical (inflammatory) stimulation. Combined single-fiber recording and psychophysical measurements in humans also show that one or a few nociceptive fibers can be active without pain and that pain does not emerge as an "all-or-nothing" response to nociceptor excitation but instead appears as the discharge frequency of several nociceptive fibers increases to within a range of total fiber activity. Furthermore, recordings from the first receiving neurons in the dorsal spinal cord show that most of them receive input from fibers with different physiological properties. Summation or integration within the CNS appears to be necessary.[1] Subsequent experiments show that the responses of CNS neurons are dramatically changed by repetitive nociceptive input so that normally ineffective innocuous stimuli now evoke neuronal discharge and pain, a process now known as *central sensitization* (see Chapter 7).

Of even greater importance, it is now evident that information from nociceptors, although normally necessary for pain, is not sufficient to account for its affective dimension. Hedonic experiences are not unique to pain, but the negative hedonic dimension of pain is not just an occasional accompaniment, it is defining and undeniably necessary. Emerging evidence that a group of subcortical and cortical structures in the medial (inner) aspect of the cerebral hemispheres participates in the elaboration of affective experiences leads to incorporating structures within the so-called limbic system into a definition of pain (see Chapter 4). This synthesis is supported by evidence that nociceptive information is widely distributed among both somatosensory and limbic structures.

The ability to image the brains of living, conscious human beings has a major impact on conceptual models of pain. Anatomical brain imaging enables the visualization of localized CNS lesions created by disease or for therapeutic reasons. It became possible to determine the effect of these lesions on the individuals in whom they appeared. The results confirm earlier, autopsy-based findings that single, focal CNS lesions do not selectively or permanently eliminate pain. Instead, pain may return or even increase, and other neurological functions may be affected. It became possible to demonstrate that the hedonic and physically discriminative components of pain were mediated by anatomically and physiologically distinct but interactive neuronal systems. With the development of functional brain imaging, it is now possible to show that subcortical and cortical components of the limbic system are active consistently during pain. Functional neuroimaging continues to guide the experimental testing of hypotheses and the development of diagnostic and therapeutic approaches to pain management.[2] It is evident that cognitive processes have a neurophysiological basis and can decrease or increase the affective quality and intensity of pain. These modulatory functions are implemented by several endogenous neurotransmitter systems that are now the targets of therapeutic drug development.

IMPLICATIONS FOR PRACTICE

This book is not about how to treat pain. However, it is important to recognize that the evolving conceptual model of pain influences practice choices. Taking account of all we are learning about pain should direct us toward improving current and future practice. The goal is to provide pain relief for as long and as specifically and as noninvasively as possible.

In practice, an early therapeutic decision is whether to focus primarily on the PNS or CNS. Focal pains will favor attention to the PNS, while multifocal or diffuse pains will favor the CNS. Both, however, demand attention.

Peripheral Nervous System

Ideally, we could ignore the complex model that includes the CNS and focus on a "labeled line" model in the PNS. The closest we can get to a labeled line to target is the nociceptor in the PNS. Unfortunately, the line begins to lose its exclusive label (or labels) upon entering the CNS. Focusing on the site of injury or disease quickly leads to considering inflammation as a target. As shown briefly in Chapter 6, inflammation is a very complex process. Fortunately, there are several anti-inflammatory agents currently in use that modify inflammation and relieve pain to a clinically significant degree. But the components of inflammation do not have pain labels. The multitude of pro-inflammatory agents offer many useful therapeutic targets[3] but also therapeutic resistance; and there are serious unwanted side effects to high degrees of inflammatory modulation. Inflammation is a necessary precursor for healing, after all, and is highly conserved through evolution.

Farther upstream, there is evidence that nociceptors and their fibers have unique ion channels that, when targeted by channel-specific antibodies delivered locally or even intravenously, reduce local inflammation and produce analgesia in mice without affecting at least one measure of motor performance.[4] This and related approaches would be a welcome improvement over the global, nonspecific effects of local anesthetics and perhaps even of systemic analgesics currently in use. However, much remains to be learned about the action of these antibodies in humans, especially in the CNS. Their local or topical application, even if limited to local pains, could possibly avoid unwanted side effects, given the distributed nature of pain mechanisms in the CNS. However, we do not know how the adaptive, plastic mechanisms in the CNS will react to a loss of nociceptive input. We now know that a suppression of nociceptive activity in the PNS or pathways in the CNS often leads to a loss of endogenous feedback control mechanisms and a return of pain or other equally unpleasant experiences. The rare cases of congenital insensitivity to pain due to mutations in the *SCNA9* gene affecting the voltage-gated sodium channel Na1.7 (see Chapter 7) suggest that normal humans could lose nociceptive input selectively and without consequences, at least for the short term. But we do not yet know how the CNS anatomy and biochemistry of these rare pain-free individuals may have changed during development to accommodate this unusual PNS physiology. We must await additional information about the short- and long-term effects of complete, selective nociceptive blockade in normal humans and in those with acute or chronic pain. Somehow, the CNS seems to adapt or maladapt to PNS changes in ways that are difficult to predict. Pain, or at least nociceptive escape or avoidance, is a highly conserved process during evolution and is likely to resist complete elimination.[5]

Central Nervous System

It is now clear that there is no labeled line for pain in the CNS. Pain emerges through the activation and interaction of central circuits that contribute to components of the pain experience. The detailed anatomy and chemistry of these circuits is being clarified by the chase for pain that continues today. As noted earlier, at least one circuit appears critical for identifying the physical properties of a painful event, others for establishing the hedonic domain, and still others for the more abstract cognitive dimensions of the experience. All these circuits function simultaneously and interact to varying degrees to create and modulate pain; and they all depend on consciousness above a preliminary level.[6] This arrangement, like the inflammatory process, has advantages and disadvantages for the treatment of pain. There are many ways to relieve pain by modifying the activity in one or more of these circuits, but given their complexity and interdependence, the chosen locus of the intervention is likely to be part of a circuit that shares a function with other circuits. Put simply, side effects may be unavoidable. That is certainly true of physical measures like focal lesions or electromagnetic stimulation as discussed earlier; it is likely to be equally true of centrally acting drugs.

Side effects are well documented effects of all the known centrally (CNS) acting analgesics. The close neurobiological link between pain and preliminary consciousness means that it is difficult, if not impossible, to affect the CNS mechanisms of pain without affecting some aspect of consciousness at the highest level. The most effective centrally acting analgesic, morphine, derives its name from Morpheus, the ancient Greek god of dreams. A primary side effect of morphine and modern opioid drugs is somnolence, often accompanied by mood change. Of course, other effects of opioids and other opiate-like analgesic drugs include their well-known addictive potential, changes in appetite, and altered basic bodily functions such as intestinal motility and respiration, to name just a few.[7] These side effects are to be expected given the wide distribution of opioid receptors throughout the brain and body. Opioid receptors are found in abundance in the thalamus, basal ganglia, upper brainstem (especially periaqueductal gray, or PAG), and hypothalamus—subcortical structures constituting preliminary consciousness as defined here.[8]

But targeting other CNS receptors such as those for serotonin and norepinephrine does not eliminate the side-effect problem. It is notable, for example, that drugs blocking the inhibitory synaptic reuptake of these neurotransmitters are effective antidepressants as well as hypalgesics for various chronic pain conditions. And gabapentin and pregabalin,[9] drugs currently used for various chronic pains and for neuropathic pain following PNS or CNS injury, act at multiple CNS sites. Their mode of action does not specifically affect the release of the inhibitory neurotransmitter gamma-aminobutyric acid (GABA) or GABA receptors. Rather, they suppress neurotransmitter release more generally by reducing the activation of a voltage-gated calcium channel that is distributed among synapses in limbic cortical areas (including cingulate cortex, the insula, and hippocampus), hypothalamus, the upper brainstem (including PAG), amygdala, and the dorsal spinal cord gray matter. Gabapentin and pregabalin appear to be most effective in reducing the excessive neuronal excitability of central sensitization, a common consequence of nerve or CNS injury—hence their use in treating neuropathic pain. Their effect on hyperexcitable states leads to their use in the treatment of anxiety disorders and as adjunctive agents for certain forms of epilepsy. Still, as might be expected from their anatomical distribution, these drugs have dose-dependent side effects including weight gain, somnolence, impaired motor coordination, and mild to moderate degrees of cognitive impairment.

If relief from mild to moderate pain is all that is necessary, acetaminophen (aka: paracetamol) has a very limited anti-inflammatory effect but does have a mild antipyretic action (via the hypothalamus) and a well-established, mild CNS hypalgesic effect due in part to an enhancement of brainstem serotonin-mediated inhibition of spinal cord nociceptive activity. This evidence is supported by the suppression of heat pain activations measured by functional magnetic resonance imaging (fMRI). There is evidence also that a metabolite of acetaminophen activates CNS cannabinoid receptors, the target of endogenous endocannabinoids, thus contributing to hypalgesia and, according to some reports, generally positive mood-altering effects as experienced with smoking marijuana. Fortunately, there are few, if any, neurological side effects if the drug is administered at the recommended dose of 1 gram every 4 to 6 hours (for adults). Liver toxicity and serious liver damage can occur following large overdoses, however.[10]

Given these limitations of CNS-based approaches to pain relief, it would seem to be futile to search for any form of side effect–free therapeutic intervention for the relief of moderate or severe pain. However, physical exercise has considerable promise for relieving many types of at least moderately painful conditions, and there is evidence that it may act at both CNS and PNS sites.[11] And there is one very ancient but "high-tech" approach that can be effective in reducing perhaps the most clinically significant component of pain: the affective dimension. It uses a selective combination of auditory frequencies that are introduced into the ear to modulate highly specific CNS circuits. When properly applied, these sounds can significantly alter circuit activity and reduce the fear and anxiety often associated with pain, especially chronic pain. They can establish realistic and acceptable expectations and help the patient cope with the pain and its cause. And they have only positive side effects! In the literature on pain treatment, this approach is often given labels such as cognitive-behavioral therapy; but more colloquially and in the real-time context of a demanding practice, it is called listening to and talking with the patient.[12]

There is an extensive literature on the application of various psychological interventions for pain. The neurophysiology of the placebo effect has been discussed earlier (see Chapter 10). Beyond that, there is evidence that more direct cognitive interventions can attenuate pain and that these effects are associated with alterations in the functional imaging activation of somatosensory and limbic structures.[13] But most practicing clinicians do not require a randomized clinical trial or functional imaging to be convinced of the therapeutic benefit of communicating about pain with a patient in pain. Many clinicians (including this one) have witnessed the relief patients experience when told, *in terms they are prepared to understand*, about the source of their neuropathic pain, about the promises and limitations of treatments, and that their pain is not caused by some unrecognized life-threatening process. Nothing allays fear and anxiety quite so well as information and understanding.

IMPLICATIONS FOR NEUROSCIENCE

The chase for pain is one very small part of the vast and complex field of neuroscience. However, the challenge to the concept of functional localization is one example of how conceptual models of pain can influence neuroscience generally. This concept has persisted during the chase for pain and remains in some form that pervades much of neuroscience today. I don't know how neuroscientists today would react to a question about how they viewed this concept. Many would probably say it is irrelevant or doesn't make sense to ask about. A few might redefine it. Others would walk away. It is almost certain that they would reject the early 20th-century model, but it is not clear what they would replace it with.[14] I suspect that many would replace the old concept with one in which localization was defined in terms of both space and time, with different neural circuits coming in and out of activity to create a continuum of experiences and responses. Certainly every experience, including pain of course, changes to varying degrees over very small and very extended periods of time. A snapshot at any given instant would show a freeze frame of neuronal activity associated with its momentary subjective and behavioral consequences. The intensity of the activity and the connectivity among neuronal groups would vary as well, giving four dimensions (space, time, intensity, and connectivity) to correlate with pain or other experiences.

Is this "pattern theory" resurrected? No. Historically, pattern theories developed to explain pain before nociceptors were discovered; they attributed pain and other sensations to different hypothetical and generally undefined patterns of impulses in PNS sensory fibers.[15] Collectively, we are not developing a new pattern theory; rather, we are replacing the old functional localization with a dynamic one that includes not simply a structure but a circuit, a group of neurons within identifiable structures and with varying degrees of activation intensity and connectivity over time. Each momentary experience and behavior would be associated with activity in specific, identifiable circuits normally driven by nociceptor activity but, in neuropathological states, also by changes in the CNS, such as those caused by stroke. The connection between neuronal activity and sensation (aka: specificity) is thus retained but in a more complex and realistic format, and it is not tied to one or a few anatomically identified structures. For neuroscience generally, this means that "function" and "location" must be defined and redefined to avoid being guided by remnants of the old phrenology.

Pain is somewhere among the structures making up the circuits discussed in this book. The chase for pain continues, leading to more refined and detailed conceptual models that challenge entrenched concepts, and it continues to influence research and the direction of medical practice.

IMPLICATIONS FOR PHILOSOPHY

We have delved into the neurobiology of consciousness as much as I care and dare to. The discussion has been largely limited to the rather obvious dependence of pain on the subcortical structures that support preliminary consciousness and the cortical structures that become activated by nociceptive input during the emergence of full consciousness. But the question remains as to whether we will ever know when the chase for pain is over, how we will recogize that event, or whether the chase can ever end at all.

I suspect that, over time and with the addition of advanced tools for investigation, we may be able to define, in exquisite anatomical, physiological, and biochemical detail, the neurobiological state that is necessary and sufficient for pain as experienced by healthy humans. This is possible because we are likely to possess the research tools needed to reveal a substantial amount of the underlying neurobiology and because humans possess language and are able to describe their experiences in great detail.[16] Physicians of the future may then be able to determine the presence, location, intensity, and other qualities of a patient's pain by inspecting and measuring the output of some currently improbable multidimensional brain scanner. That would be equivalent to reading the mind from the perspective of pain experiences. It could be useful in some special circumstances such as the vegetative state or even minimally conscious state. It would almost certainly be very expensive.

However, we do not know if the neurobiology of pain is the same for nervous systems that have been altered by injury or disease, especially if the somatosensory system is affected. The nervous system adapts to changes in the environment (memory, learning), and it changes, sometimes favorably (recovery), sometimes pathologically (e.g., central pain), in response to injury. Functions like pain may then be mediated by circuits that are different in subtle or even radical ways. As a fundamental, primordial experience, pain, like thirst, hunger, and behavioral thermoregulation, has a high priority and has evolved to resist complete elimination.

Beyond humans, we cannot be sure that the nervous systems of different animals use circuits that are similar in some recognizable way to the circuits used by healthy humans. A commonality among all animals is that their central nervous systems evolved as exploratory organs that enabled or facilitated their escape from unfavorable environments, thus favoring the development of nociceptive systems and perhaps pain or something like pain. Nonetheless, animals with different evolutionary histories can be expected to be different in several ways, and the neurobiology of nociception and pain (or its animal equivalent) may be among them.[17]

But even if we were able to identify, with microscopic and molecular precision, the physical neurobiology of pain in humans and other animals, we would still be left with the "hard problem." As noted in Chapter 11, we may never have the intellectual or investigative tools to bridge the conceptual gap between the physical and experiential worlds. The current structure of our brains may not be able to form the bridge. We may be left with only a correlative connection without the satisfying feeling of understanding that comes from translating an abstract concept into an imagined familiar experience. There is no "imagined familiar experience" of action potentials and neurotransmitter release; only their consequence is experienced. If Mozart heard the music vividly as he penned or read the notes, he would be unable, even today, to tell us how that connection was achieved; he would probably say, "It just happens." Our physicians of the distant future would give a similar response if asked to explain how a specific pattern of brain activity produces pain. This is not to say that there is no bridge between these two worlds, only that we are not equipped to understand it. We can't explain the cosmos to a sparrow.

But our conceptual limitations should not deter us from continuing the chase for pain. We see in the brief summary offered in this book that substantial practical benefits have accrued from the chase, and there is no reason to doubt that they will continue as the chase proceeds. The benefits come from the chase, not the capture. During the chase, our conceptual models, and the expectations derived from them, become more realistic— much to the benefit of neuroscience generally and of patients in pain in particular.

APPENDIX

The following is a highly distilled version of the basic mechanisms underlying the function of the mammalian nervous system; it is intended to provide a background or refresher for the non-neuroscientist's understanding of the neurobiological basis of pain research as presented in the main text.

THE NEURON

Nerve cells (neurons) in the brain generally look something like the examples shown in Figure A.1. The cell bodies of neurons like these are about 10 to 30 μm (0.01–0.03 millimeters) in diameter. The multiple dendritic branches emanating from the cell body have thousands of spines that form the receiving (input) sites for one of several different types of chemical neurotransmitters released by other neurons.

Neurons are chemical neurotransmitter factories and delivery systems. The neurotransmitter is released from the neuron by an electrical impulse (see later) that is usually generated near the junction of the cell body and the axon (the axon hillock) and transmitted along the axon to a presynaptic ending on the postsynaptic dendritic spine of a receiving neuron. Axonal length varies greatly among neurons; some axons are less than a millimeter long, but others extend these microscopic processes from human (or giraffe!) spinal cord cell bodies in the middle back through the length of the leg to the foot. The presynaptic ending of the axon and the postsynaptic membrane of the dendritic spine constitute a synapse, the site of action of chemical neurotransmitters. There are an estimated 95 to 100 billion neurons in the human central nervous system (CNS; brain, brainstem, cerebellum, and spinal cord), and for each neuron, there are thousands, in fact many thousands, of synapses. Neurons are surrounded by supporting cells (glia) that participate in neuronal metabolism, the distribution and cycling of neurotransmitters, blood-neuronal communication, and the facilitation of neuronal impulse conduction (see later).

THE ACTION POTENTIAL, A NEURAL COMMUNICATION SIGNAL

The neuron, like a battery, maintains an electrical charge across a membrane that separates the inside of the cell from the outside. Most of the energy metabolism of the brain is devoted to maintaining this charge (the membrane potential) through the continuous activity of an enzyme that keeps the intracellular concentrations of the positively charged sodium ions low and the potassium ions high relative to the extracellular space. Additional negative charges are bound to molecules that cannot cross the cell membrane; consequently, the intracellular space has a net negative charge relative to the extracellular space. As shown in Figure A.2, lowering (depolarizing) the transmembrane voltage from –70 to –55 millivolts (mV) briefly opens voltage-gated channels in the membrane, allowing an influx of sodium ion, an efflux

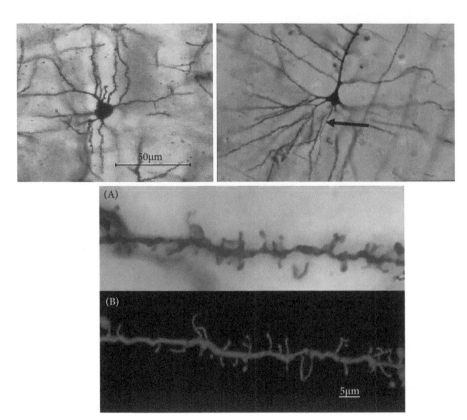

FIGURE A.1. *Upper panels* show two neurons with different shapes and patterns of dendrites radiating out from the cell body. Note *left upper panel* calibration mark of 50 microns (0.050 millimeters). *Arrow* in *right upper panel* points to the thin axon of this neuron. *Lower panels* show the detail of a dendrite with its dendritic spines; image A is from a light microscope, and image B is a three-dimensional computer reconstruction of image A. Note the calibration mark of 5 microns (0.005 millimeters).

Upper left panel from Churchill JD, Tharp JA, Wellman CL, Sengelaub DR, and Garraghty PE. Morphological correlates of injury-induced reorganization in primate somatosensory cortex. *BMC Neuroscience 5*: 43, 2004. *Upper right panel* from https://upload.wikimedia.org/wikipedia/commons/6/6d/GolgiStainedPyramidalCell.jpg. Original uploader: Cahass at https://commons.wikimedia.org/w/index.php?curid=651365. Photo by Bob Jacobs, Laboratory of Quantitative Neuromorphology Department of Psychology Colorado College. *Lower panels* from Garcia-Lopez P, Garcia-Marin V, Freire M. Three-dimensional reconstruction and quantitative study of a pyramidal cell of a Cajal histological preparation. *Journal of Neuroscience 26*: 11249–11252, 2006, with permission of the Society for Neuroscience.

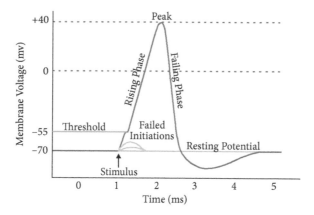

FIGURE A.2. Action potential.

From http://www.geon.us/Memory/Neuron.htm. Original by en:User:Chris 73, updated by en:User:Diberri, converted to SVG by tiZom—Own work, CC BY-SA 3.0, https://commons.wikimedia.org/w/index.php?curid=2241513.

of potassium ion, and the consequent generation of a transient (1–2 milliseconds) shift of membrane potential to a peak of +40 mV. The membrane quickly repolarizes to the negative resting potential following a slight negative overshoot. This transient voltage spike (the *action potential*) is the primary means of interneuronal communication; it propagates along the axon to the presynaptic terminal at the end of the axon where the voltage change activates mechanisms (discussed later), leading to the release of a chemical neurotransmitter onto the receptor membrane of the receiving neuron. The propagation of the action potential is made possible by the presence along the axon of voltage-gated sodium and potassium ion channels that open up as the action potential approaches and close as it passes by. The speed of action potential propagation is increased if the axon is wrapped in a glial covering (myelin) because the impulse hops between gaps in the myelin covering.

Normally, the "stimulus" shown in Figure A.2 is the release of a chemical neurotransmitter (such as the amino acid glutamate) from the presynaptic ending of another neuron onto the receiving neuron's dendritic spine or, less often, cell body (soma), producing subthreshold depolarizations or excitatory postsynaptic potentials (EPSPs), shown as "failed initiations" in Figure A.2. If many of these EPSPs are close together in time and space (on the receiving neuron's membrane), their voltage changes will add together (spatial and temporal summation), triggering an action potential in the axon of the receiving neuron. Counteracting the excitatory effect of EPSPs are inhibitory postsynaptic potentials (IPSPs), which are generated by chemical neurotransmitters like gamma-aminobutyric acid (GABA) released by nearby short-axoned neurons. IPSPs will summate just as EPSPs do. The algebraic summation of EPSPs and IPSPs over time and space on the neuronal membrane exemplifies the *integrative* capacity of the neuron.

SYNAPSES, NEUROTRANSMITTERS, AND RECEPTORS

When an action potential reaches the presynaptic ending of an axon, more voltage-gated ion channels open, allowing calcium ions to activate proteins that fuse neurotransmitter-containing vesicles to the inside of the presynaptic membrane.[1] The vesicles then release the chemical into the space (synaptic cleft) between the presynaptic and receiving (postsynaptic)

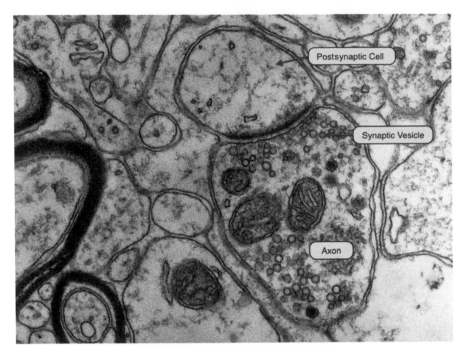

FIGURE A.3. Electron microscopic image of a synapse. An axon, with synaptic vesicles containing a neurotransmitter, is contacting the dendrite of a postsynaptic neuron. The synaptic cleft is the space between the presynaptic axon and the dendritic bouton, which has a dark postsynaptic membrane. Three axons sheathed in myelin (*dark bands*) are seen on the *left*.

Image obtained from http://medcell.med.yale.edu/systems_cell_biology/nervous_system_lab/images/synapse_em_labels.jpg, with permission of Thomas Lawrence Lentz, MD. (© 2016) Yale School of Medicine. All rights reserved.

membranes (Figure A.3). The released neurotransmitter binds to *receptors*, protein-based structures embedded in the postsynaptic membrane, that open up channels for the flow of charged ions into the postsynaptic neuron.

Excitatory receptors open up cation (positively charged ion) channels (e.g., sodium ion) to generate EPSPs; examples include receptors for glutamate, aspartate, serotonin, dopamine, noradrenaline, and acetylcholine. Inhibitory receptors open up anion (negatively charged ion) channels (e.g., chloride ion) to generate IPSPs; examples include receptors for GABA and glycine. There may be several types of receptors for each neurotransmitter, each with different postsynaptic effects. There are also postsynaptic and even presynaptic receptors for several different peptides (small chains of amino acids) found in the brain and spinal cord, including, for example, three types of receptors for opiate-like (opioid) compounds. Except for dopamine and serotonin, the distribution of receptor types does not appear to be closely linked to anatomically unique neuroanatomical pathways.

A neurotransmitter's action depends on how the postsynaptic receptor is coupled to ion channels. Some coupling is direct, rapid, and brief (1–2 milliseconds); other coupling involves the activation of intracellular proteins and is slower, of longer duration (tens or hundreds of milliseconds), and may include complex intracellular effects such as long-term changes in neuronal excitability, protein synthesis, and even gene expression. The effectiveness of a neurotransmitter is also determined by several factors such as presynaptic and postsynaptic transmembrane potentials, the action of chemicals such as peptides and nitric oxide released by the postsynaptic neuron, and the presence of enzymes that destroy and molecular transporters that recycle the transmitter. The recycling of neurotransmitters, especially glutamate, is coupled by glial cells to the ionic transport mechanisms that maintain transmembrane voltage, thus accounting for a very high percentage of the glucose-based energy metabolism of the nervous system.[2]

It is important to emphasize that these and many other modifying influences such as growth factors and hormones can profoundly increase or decrease the postsynaptic effects of an action potential at the presynaptic membrane and thus produce long-term changes in the effectiveness of synaptic transmission.

In addition to these chemical synapses, there are a few direct electrical interneuronal connections that lack a synaptic cleft and in which voltage changes and current flows occur between the fused membranes of two or more neurons. These electrical synapses may, for example, connect the dendrites of neighboring neurons with one another and facilitate the synchronized activity of groups of neurons.

THE PERIPHERAL NERVOUS SYSTEM AND CENTRAL NERVOUS SYSTEM

Peripheral nerves located in the body, head, and internal organs constitute the *peripheral nervous system* (PNS); they transmit action potentials to and from the CNS (Figure A.4). Each peripheral nerve is composed of hundreds of thousands of nerve fibers, which are the action potential conductors of individual neurons.

The *somatic peripheral nervous system* (sPNS) is comprised of neurons that communicate sensory information and motor commands between the CNS and the skin, muscle, and bones of the body. Output command (or "motor") neurons of the sPNS send their axons directly to muscles that move parts of the body that are under voluntary control and can be trained or conditioned; the neurotransmitter to these muscles is acetylcholine.

Internal organs, such as the heart, lungs, blood vessels, bowel, bladder, and glandular tissues, communicate with the CNS via the *autonomic peripheral nervous system* (aPNS).[3] Output command neurons of the aPNS affect internal and glandular organs indirectly, through synaptic connections with clusters of neurons called *ganglia* located either just outside the spinal cord or near the target organ. Voluntary control and conditioning of aPNS targets is very limited, as suggested by the term "autonomic."[4] The predominant neurotransmitters acting on internal organs are norepinephrine (the *sympathetic* aPNS) and acetylcholine (the *parasympathetic* aPNS). Some functions and control of the sympathetic and parasympathetic aPNS are discussed in subsequent paragraphs.

Nerve fibers of the sPNS and aPNS are located together in most peripheral nerves. PNS nerve fibers with a *motor* or *secretory* function have cell bodies in the spinal cord or brainstem of the CNS. PNS nerve fibers with a *sensory* function have cell bodies in sensory ganglia located just outside the spinal cord or brainstem, or within specialized sensory organs like the eye, ear, tongue, or nose. The cell bodies of sensory neurons do not have dendrites like the neurons depicted in Figure A.1; rather, they have axons with a *peripheral* branch extending from the cell body into the tissues of the body and internal organs and a *central* branch going from the cell body into the spinal cord or brainstem. The peptides *substance P* and *calcitonin gene–related peptide* (CGRP) are neurotransmitters released by central branches in the spinal

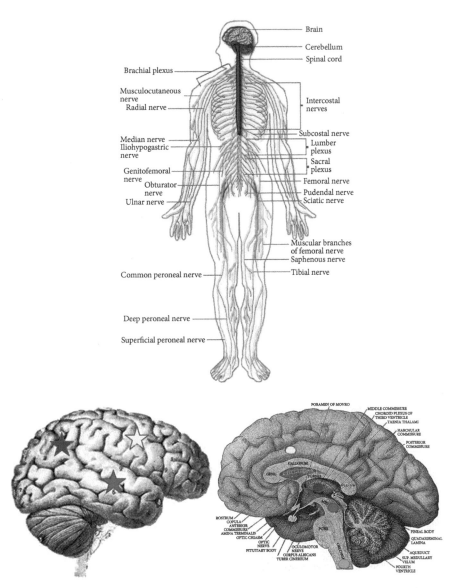

FIGURE A.4. The peripheral nervous system (PNS) and central nervous system (PNS). *Please don't be distracted by the many labels in this figure,* which is intended only to provide a very basic reminder of the overall architecture of the human nervous system as a guide to the main text in this book. The *upper panel* depicts the CNS in *red* and the somatic part of the peripheral nervous system (sPNS) in *blue*. Some of the nerves shown here contain fibers of the autonomic nervous system (aPNS, not shown) also. The figurine conveys the impression that the modestly sized CNS receives and integrates an enormous amount of sensory information from the body (and internal organs), all in addition to inputs from visual, auditory, olfactory, and gustatory sources. The *colored stars* in the *left lower panel* are placed over the frontal (*yellow*), parietal (*red*), and temporal (*blue*) lobes of a right hemisphere, the medial (or inner) surface of which is shown in the *right lower panel*. The *colored circles* in that panel are placed over the upper (cervical) part of the spinal cord (*green*), the upper brainstem and midbrain (*blue*), the thalamus (*red*), and the cortex of the cingulate gyrus (*yellow*). The hypothalamus lies between the thalamus and the pituitary body, which can be seen hanging like a bell from cord and brainstem by sensory nerve fibers with peripheral endings (*receptors*) that are excited by stimuli that are normally painful.

The sensory input from the aPNS to the spinal cord and brainstem partially overlaps the sensory input from the sPNS. In fact, there is a substantial degree of synaptic convergence of internal organ (e.g., visceral) and somatic sensory input onto single neurons at several sites within the CNS. Nonetheless, under normal circumstances, we are only intermittently aware of a few visceral sensations (e.g., bladder and bowel) but are continually aware of sensations from the skin and muscles of the body. Under pathological conditions, however (e.g., heart attack, gallbladder inflammation, kidney stone), the input from visceral sensory fibers may be great enough to be perceived as pain within or near the body area that shares sensory innervation with the affected organ (e.g., pain in the left arm or chest during a heart attack). The neurophysiological mechanisms underlying this *referred pain* are still being investigated.[5]

Neurons, the axonal pathways connecting them, and the synapses between them are organized into specialized, complex pathways within the CNS.

The *spinal cord* is devoted to receiving and sending action potentials via PNS neurons innervating the body (sPNS) and internal organs (aPNS). The cell bodies of spinal cord motor and sensory neurons are located in the center of the spinal cord (the *gray matter*); their axons are found in the surrounding *white matter* (so named because many axons are ensheathed by glial cells in whitish myelin), which connects the spinal cord with CNS structures located above them. The *brainstem* differs from the spinal cord in that, in addition to serving somatic sensory, motor, and autonomic functions of structures in the head, it also receives sensory information for taste, hearing, and the sense of body position or motion in space (vestibular function). Sensory inputs to the CNS from the optic, auditory, olfactory, and gustatory nerves are activated by receptors specialized to respond to extracorporeal environmental changes and do not directly excite synaptic connections in the spinal cord.

The *thalamus* is composed of several distinctive clusters (called nuclei) of nerve cells that receive synaptic inputs from the axons of sensory neurons of the spinal cord and brainstem, distribute this information to specialized areas of the cerebral cortex, and receive synaptic inputs from those same cortical areas. Thalamocortical connections are organized and separated according to sensory (visual, auditory, somatic, and gustatory), motor (e.g., face, arm, leg), and associative or cognitive functions. This anatomical and physiological arrangement allows the thalamus to monitor and control these functions of the cerebral cortex. Not all thalamic neurons send axons to the cerebral cortex; many are short-axoned inhibitory interneurons that also receive spinal, brainstem, and cortical synapses. Information that is

---

FIGURE A.4. Continued

the pituitary stalk in front of the brainstem. The basal ganglia (not shown) are located in front of the thalamus and, together with the thalamus, constitute the major channels of communication with the cerebral cortex. The cerebellum is located between the brainstem and the occipital (back or posterior) lobe of the brain.

Upper panel from https://wikimedia.org/wikipedia/commons/b/ba/Nervous_system_diagram.png. By □~Persian Poet Gal (Own work) [Public domain], via Wikimedia Commons. *Left lower panel from* https://comons.wikimedia.org/wiki/File:PSM_V46_D167_Outer_surface_of_the_human_brain.jpg, author unknown. *Right lower panel* by Henry Vandyke Carter—Henry Gray (1918). *Anatomy of the Human Body,* Bartleby.com: *Gray's Anatomy,* Plate 715, public domain, https://wikimedia.org/wikipedia/commons/d/d7/Gray715.png.

critical for the perception of temperature and pain reaches the thalamus primarily through the *spinothalamic tract* of the ventrolateral spinal cord and its counterpart in the brainstem.

The *basal ganglia* are neuronal structures located near the base of the brain, in front of the thalamus, and within the inner (middle) aspect of each cerebral hemisphere.[6] The main structures of the basal ganglia include the caudate nucleus and putamen (comprising the striatum), and the adjacent output structure, the globus pallidus. Various authors include other anatomically related brain and upper brainstem structures (such as the substantia nigra) within the basal ganglia; among these, the *amygdala*, located at the tips of the temporal lobes, and the *nucleus accumbens*, located adjacent to the caudate nucleus, are likely especially relevant for participating in the generation and modulation of pain because of their neurotransmitter content (dopamine, opioids) and direct connections with the hypothalamus, limbic cortex, and upper brainstem. The basal ganglia receive inputs from a wide range of sources, predominantly the cerebral cortex, middle or inner thalamus, amygdala, and upper brainstem. Neurons that respond exclusively or differentially to noxious stimuli are found, sometimes in high proportions, in several basal ganglia structures. Basal ganglia outputs are directed primarily back to the cerebral cortex and outer or lateral thalamus. Receptors for dopamine, opioid, acetylcholine, GABA, acetylcholine, and glutamate neurotransmission are found within this neuronal group. Excitatory influences are often implemented by inhibiting inhibitory neurons (disinhibition). Many authors recognize three functional divisions of the basal ganglia: sensorimotor, associative (or cognitive), and limbic (or affective and emotional), depending on the communicating territories of the cerebral cortex. Summarizing the function of the basal ganglia is difficult because of the anatomical, physiological, and biochemical complexity of this group of neurons. One overview is that *the basal ganglia form a neuronal hub that integrates information from the limbic cortex, thalamus, and brainstem to modulate interactions between the thalamus and cerebral cortex.*

The *hypothalamus*, as the name indicates, is made up of small clusters of neurons located just below the thalamus; it receives input from the spinal cord (spinohypothalamic tract),[7] multiple structures in the brainstem, and the cerebral cortex, primarily the temporal and frontal lobes. Despite its relatively small size, the hypothalamus is a major controller of all vital autonomic and endocrine functions including temperature, heart rate, blood pressure, fluid balance, and the secretion of multiple hormones that are critical for reproduction and combating infection and injury. The hypothalamus controls some hormonal functions by regulating the secretion of hormones from the pituitary gland, which is enclosed in a bony cup at the base of the skull.

The immediate response to environmental changes is mediated through hypothalamic control of the sympathetic and parasympathetic aPNS mentioned previously. In maintaining normal internal body functions (homeostasis), the sympathetic and parasympathetic systems function together as a highly integrated mechanism. The parasympathetic aPNS (using the neurotransmitter acetylcholine) slows heart rate and generally promotes several secretory (salivation, tearing) and waste elimination (bladder, bowel) functions. The sympathetic component of the aPNS (using norepinephrine as a neurotransmitter) is perhaps most important for its association with pain; it recruits responses that are appropriate for defending against attacks or perceived threat of attack. When fully employed in extreme circumstances, the sympathetic aPNS accelerates heart and respiratory rate, raises blood pressure, increases muscle blood flow, decreases skin blood flow, and dilates the pupils. These responses are typically accompanied by feelings of a desire to act or of fear or anger. As discussed elsewhere in this book, the hypothalamus is an important component of both the objective and subjective aspects of pain.

All parts of the CNS shown in Figure A.4 are connected with one another either directly through one synapse or indirectly through multiple synapses. The long connections linking the major CNS components together are excitatory. Glutamate is the most common CNS neurotransmitter; acetylcholine, serotonin, norepinephrine, and a variety of peptides are also important. Inhibition is achieved by the excitation of short-axoned neurons (interneurons) that typically release GABA or glycine as the neurotransmitters.

In thinking about the neurophysiology of pain, it is important to realize that, in normal humans, action potentials are continuously generated in the spinal cord, brainstem, and brain, simultaneously ascending to and descending from many CNS structures during wakefulness and sleep. The brain is silent only in death.

CEREBROSPINAL FLUID, THE MENINGES, AND THE BLOOD-BRAIN BARRIER

The CNS is a physically soft electrochemical organ that, during the course of evolution, acquired protection from potentially harmful physical and chemical influences in the external and immediately surrounding environments. The protective system that emerged has enabled survival but also limits our ability to manipulate CNS function—and to treat pain, for example. This is why it is important to have some understanding of what is called the *blood-brain barrier* (BBB) as part of the story of chasing pain.[8]

The entire human CNS is bathed and cushioned by approximately 150 milliliters of clear, watery cerebrospinal fluid (CSF) that is produced primarily by a specialized, blood-rich tissue (*choroid plexus*) located in the chamber-like ventricles deep within each cerebral hemisphere and the brainstem. CSF is produced by the active (energy-requiring) transport of water and of sodium, potassium, and bicarbonate ions at a rate of 500 mL/day; it is reabsorbed at the same rate into the blood by cells located near venous blood vessels in a thin, spider web–like sheet of tissue (hence the name *arachnoid membrane*) that covers the CNS. The arachnoid membrane is itself covered by a much thicker, stronger, and more protective fibrous membrane (hence the name *dura mater* or simply *dura*). The arachnoid membrane and the dura mater make up the *meninges* that cover the CNS. There are chemically and mechanically sensitive nerve endings with receptors (nociceptors) in the dura (but not the CNS), primarily near meningeal blood vessels. Excitation of these nociceptors by inflammation sends action potentials to the brainstem of the CNS, usually producing a severe headache that may signal the presence of meningitis or hemorrhage.

The composition of the CSF is quite different from that of the blood because of the filtering and molecular transport activity of cells in the choroid plexus and the walls of CNS capillaries. These tissues make up a barrier (the BBB), which includes the interposed blood-CSF barrier (BCSFB) of the choroid plexus; it impedes the entry of water-soluble (hydrophilic) molecules and ions while favoring the passage of lipid-soluble (lipophilic) substances into the CSF. The barrier function is partly passive and attributable to the physical properties of the cellular and membrane elements of the BBB.[9] Thus, large, water-soluble protein molecules and smaller amino acid chains (peptides) are generally excluded by this passive filtering function. Neurotransmitters, which are produced by CNS neurons, are largely excluded from entering the CSF from the blood. Low-molecular-weight steroids, such as cortisol and the sex hormones, have access to the CSF and CNS only if not bound to a large protein such as albumin. Glial cells in the CNS produce steroids, but these act only locally within the CNS to modulate neuronal excitability through their action on neurotransmitter receptors.

There are specific, energy-demanding transport mechanisms that operate in parallel with passive filters to actively transport molecules between the CSF and the blood, thus permitting the entry of molecules that might otherwise be excluded because of their physical properties.[10] For example, glucose, the water-soluble and critical CNS energy source, is actively transported into the CSF. Consequently, when the BBB is impaired by disease or injury, CSF protein concentration may be abnormally high at the same time that glucose concentration is abnormally low. Some amino acids, including components of certain neurotransmitters, are actively transported from the blood to the CNS. The filtering action of the BBB is not uniformly distributed, however; it is normally modified at CNS locations such as the hypothalamus and at some locations in the brainstem, allowing oxygen, carbon dioxide, hormones, and inflammatory signaling molecules to affect the activity of CNS neuronal circuits, including those participating in the generation of pain.

The activity and function of the BBB is an important determinant of the effectiveness of drugs for treating pain. Because of the combined passive and active mechanisms that form the BBB, an a priori prediction of drug penetration into the CNS is difficult; consequently, animal experiments and human clinical trials are required. Drugs that produce analgesia primarily by reducing the inflammatory excitation of nociceptors, such as aspirin and other hydrophilic nonsteroidal anti-inflammatory drugs, need not pass through the BBB to be effective. There is evidence that a clinically significant component of the analgesia produced by the free, protein-*unbound* form of these compounds is due to their effect on some CNS pain mechanisms, but this is likely to be less important than their well-known and robust attenuation of the excitation of nociceptors by inflammatory mediators.[11] In contrast, the potent analgesic effect of lipophilic opioid compounds such as morphine and codeine is known to depend strongly on their activation of opioid receptors and their associated circuitry in the CNS (discussed in the main text). The development of highly lipophilic BBB-penetrating drugs such as fentanyl and remifentanil was intended to facilitate this CNS effect.[12] Nonetheless, there are opioid receptors in tissues outside the CNS, and there is some clinical evidence that these could be effective targets for opioid analgesics if their CNS side effects, such as sedation and gastrointestinal dysfunction, could be avoided by restricting their penetration of the BBB.[13]

NOTES

Introduction

1. Borsook D. Neurological diseases and pain. *Brain 135*: 320–344, 2012.
2. Gaskin DJ, and Richard P. The economic costs of pain in the United States. *Journal of Pain 13*: 715–724, 2012. The average cost of a single, prime-time, 30s TV advertisement was approximately $100,000 in 2010 (www.adweek.com). For a detailed discussion of the magnitude of pain as a medical, economic, and societal problem, see: Institute of Medicine. *Relieving Pain in America: A Blueprint for Transforming Prevention, Care, Education, and Research*. Washington, DC: National Academies Press, 2011, p. 364; Forman J. *A Nation in Pain*. New York: Oxford University Press, 2014, p. 464.
3. For an amusing example of how conceptual models affect daily living, see: Kempton W. Two theories of home heat control. *Cognitive Science 10*: 90, 1986. (Reference courtesy of Lyman Casey, Ph.D., www.centralis.com.)

Chapter 1

1. Livingston WK. *Pain and Suffering*. Seattle: IASP Press, 1998, pp. 103–117.
2. Melzack R, and Loeser JD. Phantom body pain in paraplegics: Evidence for a central "pattern generating mechanism" for pain. *Pain 4*: 195–210, 1978.
3. *Analgesia* means the absence of pain; the preservation of consciousness is generally assumed. *Hypalgesia* is the medical term for reduced pain; *anesthesia* is the absence of all body sensations and usually assumes an unconscious state (see *Dorland's Illustrated Medical Dictionary*, 32nd edition. Philadelphia: W.B. Saunders, 2011).
4. Bowers A. *Mandan Social and Ceremonial Organization*. Lincoln: University of Nebraska Press, 2004, p. 407.
5. Marshall W. *The Therapeutic Experience of Being Suspended by Your Skin*. In: *The Atlantic*. The Atlantic Monthly Group, September 2012; http://www.theatlantic.com/health/print/2012/09/thetherapeuticexperienceofbeingsuspendedbyyourskin/262644/.
6. Pernick MS. The calculus of suffering in nineteenth-century surgery. *Hastings Center Report 13*: 26–36, 1983. Ether was introduced as a general anesthetic in October of 1846, and cocaine was first used as a local anesthetic in ophthalmological surgery in 1884 (Sabatowski R, Schafer D, Kasper SM, Brunsch H, and Radbruch L. Pain treatment: A historical overview. *Current Pharmaceutical Design 10*: 701–716, 2004.).
7. Hayot E. *The Hypothetical Mandarin: Sympathy, Modernity, and Chinese Pain*. New York: Oxford University Press, 2009, p. 278.
8. The Acupuncture Anesthesia Study Group was sponsored by the Committee on Scholarly Communication with the People's Republic of China of the American Council of Learned Societies, the National Academy of Sciences, and the Social Science Research Council, all approved by the Governing Board of the National Research Council (United States).

9. *Acupuncture Anesthesia in the People's Republic of China*. Washington, DC: National Academy of Sciences Press, 1976.
10. See: Chapters 1 and 2 in: *Acupuncture Anesthesia*, US Department of Health, Education, and Welfare, Publication No. (NIH) 75-784, US Gov't Printing Office, Washington, DC, 1975; Unschuld PU, *Medicine in China: A History of Ideas*, University of California Press, 1985, pp. 92–99.
11. Taylor K. *Chinese Medicine in Early Communist China, 1945–63.* New York: RoutledgeCu rzon, 2005.
12. Reston J. *Now, About My Operation in Peking, The New York Times*, July 26, 1971, p. 1.
13. Video clips of three surgeries (thyroid adenectomy, ovarian cystectomy, and pulmonary lobectomy) performed with acupuncture only are available on the following website: https://books.google.com/books?id=UjQrAAAAYAAJ&lpg=PR1&dq=inauthor%3A %22American%20Acupuncture%20Anesthesia%20Study%20Group%22&pg=PP1#v=on epage&q&f=false.
14. Personal notes from tape recordings made in China by the author and transcribed by the late Catherine Corson, Executive Secretary, Department of Physiology, University of Michigan, Ann Arbor, 1974.
15. http://www.acuwatch.org/general/taub.shtml
16. Unschuld PU, *Medicine in China: A History of Ideas*, University of California Press, 1985, pp. 360–366.
17. Taylor K. *Chinese Medicine in Early Communist China, 1945–63,* New York: RoutledgeCu rzon, 2005.
18. Wang SM, et al. Acupuncture analgesia: II. Clinical considerations. *Anesthesia and Analgesia 106*: 611–21, 2008.; Han JS, Acupuncture analgesia: Areas of consensus and controversy. *Pain 152*: S41–S48, 2011.

Chapter 2

1. From definition 1b of *Webster's Third New International Dictionary* (unabridged), Springfield, MA, 1971: "Involving the psychological range of feelings from pleasant to unpleasant."
2. Today, the IASP has nearly 8000 members distributed among 133 countries. More than half of all IASP members are self-identified clinicians, and nearly a third are engaged in either clinical or basic scientific research, much of which is published in *Pain*, the peer-reviewed journal of the IASP. IASP funds support pain-related education and training worldwide with an emphasis on developing countries. John would be deservedly proud of this organization today.
3. The history of this directive for the healing professions is thoroughly discussed in: Smith CM. Origin and uses of primum non nocere—above all, do no harm! *Journal of Clinical Pharmacology 45*: 371–377, 2005.
4. Slightly more than 30,000 have attended the annual meetings from 2007 through 2016 (http://www.sfn.org/annual-meeting/past-and-future-annual-meetings/annual-meeting-attendance-statistics).
5. Heinbecker P, and Bishop GH. The mechanism of painful sensations. *Proceedings of the Association for Research on Nervous and Mental Disease 15*: 226–238, 1934.
6. Bessou P, and Perl ER. Response of cutaneous sensory units with unmyelinated fibers to noxious stimuli. *Journal of Neurophysiology 32*: 1025–1043, 1969; Burgess PR, and Perl ER. Myelinated afferent fibers responding specifically to noxious stimulation of the skin.

Journal of Physiology 190: 541–562, 1967. In a broad-ranging review of the early and contemporary history of pain research, Perl discusses early theories (pattern vs. specificity) and the experiments that led to the discovery of nociceptors: Perl ER. Pain mechanisms: A commentary on concepts and issues. *Progress in Neurobiology 94*: 20–38, 2011.

7. Melzack R, and Wall PD. Pain mechanisms: A new theory. *Science* 150: 971–979, 1965. This publication, probably more than any other, initiated the contemporary surge in research on both basic scientific and clinical aspects of pain.

8. Livingston WK. *Pain and Suffering*. Seattle: IASP Press, 1998, p. 245.; Livingston WK. *Pain Mechanisms*. New York: Macmillan, 1943, p. 251. Livingston, a neurosurgeon, was convinced by his clinical experience that the prevailing simplistic model of pain mechanisms could not be correct. He offered many clinical examples of how the perception of pain was often poorly related to the degree of tissue injury.

Chapter 3

1. For a detailed review of the history of the location of functions in the nervous system, see: Finger S, *Origins of Neuroscience: A History of Explorations into Brain Function*, Chapters 1–4. New York: Oxford University Press, 1994, pp. 3–62.

2. The following sources have more information about early theories of pain and pain treatments: Rey R. *History of Pain*. Paris: La Decouverte, 1993, p. 408; Sabatowski R, et al. Pain treatment: A historical overview. *Current Pharmaceutical Design 10*: 701–716, 2004; Zimmermann M. The history of pain concepts and treatment before IASP, Chapter 1. In: Merskey H, Loeser JD, Dubner R (Eds.), *Paths of Pain*. Seattle: IASP Press, 2005, pp. 1–21; Perl ER. Pain mechanisms: A commentary on concepts and issues. *Progress in Neurobiology 94*: 20–38, 2011.

3. Finger S, *Origins of Neuroscience: A History of Explorations into Brain Function*, Chapters 1–4. New York: Oxford University Press, 1994, p. 156.

4. Translation of De la transmission des impressions sensitives par la moelle epiniere, *Compt Rend Soc Biol 1*: 192–194, 1849, In: Wilkins RH, and Brody I (Eds.), *Neurological Classics*. New York: Johnson Reprint Corporation, 1973, pp. 49–50.

5. Tattersall R, and Turner B. Brown-Sequard and his syndrome. *Lancet 356*: 61–63, 2000.

6. Spiller WG, and Martin E. The treatment of persistent pain of organic origin in the lower part of the body by division of the anterolateral column of the spinal cord. *Journal of the American Medical Association 58*: 1489–1492, 1912; Cadwalader WB, and Sweet JE. Experimental work on the function of the anterolateral column of the spinal cord. *Journal of the American Medical Association 58*: 1490–1493, 1912.

7. Heinbecker P, and Bishop GH. The mechanism of painful sensations. *Proceedings of the Association for Research on Nervous and Mental Disease 15*: 226–238, 1934.

8. The following sources provide more information and references about postcordotomy pain and return of pain: Livingston WK. *Pain Mechanisms*. New York: Plenum Press, 1976, pp. 24–25; Noordenbos W. *Pain*. Amsterdam: Elsevier, 1959, pp. 165–172; Villanueva L, and Nathan PW. Multiple pain pathways. In: Devor M, Rowbotham M, and Wiesenfeld-Hallin Z (Eds.), *Proceedings of the 9th World Congress on Pain*. Scattle: IASP Press, 2000, pp. 371–386; White JC, and Sweet WH. *Pain: Its Mechanisms and Neurosurgical Control*. Springfield, IL: C.C. Thomas, 1955, pp. 240–286; White JC, and Sweet WH. *Pain and the Neurosurgeon. A Forty-Year Experience*. Springfield, IL: C.C. Thomas, 1969; Cowie RA, and Hitchcock ER. The late results of antero-lateral cordotomy for pain relief. *Acta Neurochirurgica 64*: 39–50, 1982; Lahuerta J, Bowsher D, Lipton S, and Buxton PH.

Percutaneous cervical cordotomy: A review of 181 operations on 146 patients with a study on the location of "pain fibers" in the C-2 spinal cord segment of 29 cases. *Journal of Neurosurgery 80*: 975–985, 1994; Nagaro T, Adachi N, Tabo E, Kimura S, Arai T, and Dote K. New pain following cordotomy: Clinical features, mechanisms, and clinical importance. *Journal of Neurosurgery 95*: 425–431, 2001; Cetas JS, Saedi T, and Burchiel KJ. Destructive procedures for the treatment of nonmalignant pain: A structured literature review. *Journal of Neurosurgery 109*: 389–404, 2008.

9. Vierck CJ Jr, and Light AR. Allodynia and hyperalgesia within dermatomes caudal to a spinal cord injury in primates and rodents. *Progress in Brain Research 129*: 411–428, 2000; Vierck CJ Jr, Siddall P, and Yezierski RP. Pain following spinal cord injury: Animal models and mechanistic studies. *Pain 89*: 1–5, 2000; Weng HR, Lee JI, Lenz FA, Schwartz A, Vierck C, Rowland L, and Dougherty PM. Functional plasticity in primate somatosensory thalamus following chronic lesion of the ventral lateral spinal cord. *Neuroscience 101*: 393–401, 2000; Liang L, and Mendell LM. Bilateral transient changes in thalamic nucleus ventroposterior lateralis after thoracic hemisection in the rat. *Journal of Neurophysiology 110*: 942–951, 2013.

10. Hitchcock ER. Stereotactic cervical myelotomy. *Journal of Neurology, Neurosurgery, and Psychiatry 33*: 224–230, 1970; Nauta HJW, Soukup VM, Fabian RH, Lin JT, Grady JJ, Williams CGA, Campbell GA, Westlund KN, and Willis WD Jr. Punctate midline myelotomy for the relief of visceral cancer pain. *Journal of Neurosurgery 92*: 125–130, 2000.

11. Noordenbos W, and Wall PD. Diverse sensory functions with an almost totally divided spinal cord: A case of spinal cord transection with preservation of part of one anterolateral quadrant. *Pain 2*: 197–198, 1976; Wall PD, and Noordenbos W. Sensory functions which remain in man after complete transection of dorsal columns. *Brain 100*: 641–653, 1977.

12. In the decade after Issaquah, an elegant, detailed study of a patient with a complete surgical interruption of the fibers (corpus callosum) connecting the cerebral hemispheres showed that pain could be perceived via *uncrossed* spinal pathways when high intensity stimuli were used. Stein BE, Price DD, and Gazzaniga MS. Pain perception in a man with total corpus callosum transection. *Pain 38*: 51–56, 1989.

13. Russell WR. Transient disturbances following gunshot wounds of the head. *Brain 68*: 79–97, 1945; Marshall J. Sensory disturbances in cortical wounds with special reference to pain. *Journal of Neurology, Neurosurgery, and Psychiatry 14*: 187–204, 1951.

14. Lighthall JW, Goshgarian HG, and Pinderski CR. Characterization of axonal injury produced by controlled cortical impact. *Journal of Neurotrauma 7*: 65–76, 1990.

15. Vierck CJ, Whitsel BL, Favorov OV, Brown AW, and Tommerdahl M. Role of primary somatosensory cortex in the coding of pain. *Pain 154*: 334–344, 2013; Chen LM, Dillenburger BC, Wang F, Friedman RM, and Avison MJ. High-resolution functional magnetic resonance imaging mapping of noxious heat and tactile activations along the central sulcus in New World monkeys. *Pain 152*: 522–532, 2011.

16. Knecht S, Kunesch E, and Schnitzler A. Parallel and serial processing of haptic information in man: Effects of parietal lesions on sensorimotor hand function. *Neuropsychologia 34*: 669–687, 1996.

17. Ramirez LF, and Levin AB. Pain relief after hypophysectomy. *Neurosurgery 14*: 499–504, 1984; Lipton S. Neurodestructive procedures in the management of cancer pain. *Journal of Pain and Symptom Management 2*: 219–228, 1987.

Chapter 4

1. Sherrington CS. Qualitative difference of spinal reflex corresponding with qualitative difference of cutaneous stimulus. *Journal of Physiology 30*: 39–46, 1903; Sherrington CS, and Laslett EE. Observations on some spinal reflexes and the interconnection of spinal segments. *Journal of Physiology 29*: 58–96, 1903; Woodworth RS, and Sherrington CS. A pseudaffective reflex and its spinal path. *Journal of Physiology 31*: 234–243, 1904.

2. The historical background of these experiments and their significance for understanding the autonomic nervous system can be found in: Cannon WB. *Bodily Changes in Pain, Hunger, Fear and Rage.* New York Appleton-Century Co., 1929, p. 404.

3. Bard P. A diencephalic mechanism for the expression of rage with special reference to the sympathetic nervous system. *American Journal of Physiology 84*: 490–515, 1928.

4. Papez JW. A proposed mechanism of emotion. *Archives of Neurological Psychiatry 38*: 725–743, 1937.

5. Ibid. 728.

6. MacLean PD. Psychosomatic disease and the "visceral brain." *Psychosomatic Medicine 11*: 338–353, 1949. Maclean PD. The limbic system ("visceral brain") and emotional behavior. *AMA Archives of Neurology and Psychiatry 73*: 130–134, 1955; MacLean PD. Visceral functions of the nervous system. *Annual Review of Physiology 19*: 397–416, 1957. The hippocampus and cingulate cortex are the key cortical structures in MacLean's definition of "limbic system." Several connected subcortical structures are included in the definition; these include the hypothalamus and "parts of the basal ganglia" (MacLean, 1955, p. 130). The inclusion of the basal ganglia has important implications for understanding the neural mechanisms of the affective component of pain discussed later in this book.

7. For a review of this evidence, see: Berridge KC. Measuring hedonic impact in animals and infants: Microstructure of affective taste reactivity patterns. *Neuroscience and Biobehavioral Reviews 24*: 173–198, 2000; Devinsky O, Morrell MJ, and Vogt BA. Contributions of anterior cingulate cortex to behaviour. *Brain 118*: 279–306, 1995; Vogt BA. Pain and emotion interactions in subregions of the cingulate gyrus. *Nature Reviews Neuroscience 6*: 533–544, 2005. Recent evidence supporting a modification and further refinement of the original limbic system concept is discussed later in this book (see Chapter 11).

8. Mehler WR, Feferman ME, and Nauta WJH. Ascending axon degeneration following anterolateral cordotomy: An experimental study in the monkey. *Brain 83*: 718–750, 1960; Nauta WJH. Hippocampal projections and related neural pathways to the midbrain in the cat. *Brain 81*: 319–340, 1958.

9. Jones EG. *The Thalamus.* New York: Plenum Press, 1985, pp. 5–8.

10. Mountcastle VB. The columnar organization of the neocortex. *Brain 120*: 701–722, 1997; Poggio GF, and Mountcastle VB. The functional properties of ventrobasal thalamic neurons studied in unanesthetized monkeys. *Journal of Neurophysiology 26*: 775–806, 1963; Raldolph M, and Semmes J. Behavioral consequences of selective subtotal ablations in the postcentral gyrus of Macaca mulatta. *Brain Research 70*: 55–70, 1974; Semmes J, Porter L, and Randolph MC. Further studies of anterior postcentral lesions in monkeys. *Cortex 10*: 55–68, 1974; LaMotte RH, and Mountcastle VB. Disorders in somesthesis following lesions of parietal lobe. *Journal of Neurophysiology 42*: 400–419, 1979; Kenshalo DR Jr, and Isensee O. Responses of primate S1 cortical neurons to noxious stimuli. *Journal of Neurophysiology 50*: 1479–1496, 1983; Bushnell MC, Duncan GH, and Tremblay N. Thalamic VPM nucleus in the behaving monkey. I. Multimodal and discriminative properties of thermosensitive neurons. *Journal of Neurophysiology 69*: 739–752, 1993;

Apkarian AV, and Shi T. Squirrel monkey lateral thalamus. I. Somatic nociresponsive neurons and their relation to spinothalamic terminals. *Journal of Neuroscience 14*: 6779–6795, 1994; Kim JS. Patterns of sensory abnormality in cortical stroke: Evidence for a dichotomized sensory system. *Neurology 68*: 174–180, 2007; Moulton EA, Keaser ML, Gullapalli RP, and Greenspan JD. Regional intensive and temporal patterns of functional MRI activation distinguishing noxious and innocuous contact heat. *Journal of Neurophysiology 93*: 2183–2193, 2005; Moulton EA, Pendse G, Becerra LR, and Borsook D. BOLD responses in somatosensory cortices better reflect heat sensation than pain. *Journal of Neuroscience 32*: 6024–6031, 2012; Vierck CJ, Whitsel BL, Favorov OV, Brown AW, and Tommerdahl M. Role of primary somatosensory cortex in the coding of pain. *Pain 154*: 334–344, 2013; Knecht S, Kunesch E, and Schnitzler A. Parallel and serial processing of haptic information in man: Effects of parietal lesions on sensorimotor hand function. *Neuropsychologia 34*: 669–687, 1996.

11. Casey KL. Unit analysis of nociceptive mechanisms in the thalamus of the awake squirrel monkey. *Journal of Neurophysiology 29*: 727–750, 1966; Bushnell MC, and Duncan GH. Sensory and affective aspects of pain perception: Is medial thalamus restricted to emotional issues? *Experimental Brain Research 78*: 415–418, 1989. (These investigators showed that, in the monkey, some medial thalamic neurons respond to small changes in noxious temperatures applied to the skin; however, these neurons are insensitive to body location, and their responses are attenuated by distraction and sedation. The authors suggest that the thermal responses may encode the affective intensity of pain.)

For a critical discussion of these and related issues, see: Willis WD, and Westlund KN. Neuroanatomy of the pain system and of the pathways that modulate pain. *Journal of Clinical Neurophysiology 14*: 2–31, 1997; Willis WD Jr, Zhang X, Honda CN, and Giesler GJ Jr. A critical review of the role of the proposed VMpo nucleus in pain. *Journal of Pain 3*: 79–94, 2002.

12. Bogousslavsky J, Regli F, and Uske A. Thalamic infarcts: Clinical syndromes, etiology, and prognosis. *Neurology 38*: 837–848, 1988; Swartz RH, and Black SE. Anterior-medial thalamic lesions in dementia: Frequent, and volume dependently associated with sudden cognitive decline. *Journal of Neurology, Neurosurgery and Psychiatry 77*: 1307–1312, 2006.

13. Vertes RP, Linley SB, and Hoover WB. Limbic circuitry of the midline thalamus. *Neuroscience and Biobehavioral Reviews 54*: 89–107, 2015.

14. Moruzzi G, and Magoun HW. Brain stem reticular formation and activation of the EEG. *Electroencephalography and Clinical Neurophysiology 1*: 455–473, 1949; French JD, Verzeano M, and Magoun HW. An extralemniscal sensory system in the brain. *AMA Archives of Neurology and Psychiatry 69*: 505–518, 1953; Nauta WJH, and Kuypers HGJM. Some ascending pathways in the brain stem reticular formation of the cat. In: Jasper HH, and Proctor LD (Eds.), *Reticular Formation of the Brain*. Boston: Little, Brown, 1958, pp. 3–30; Ramon-Moliner E, and Nauta WJH. The isodendritic core of the brain stem. *Journal of Comparative Neurology 126*: 311–336, 1966. See also: Craig AD Jr, and Burton H. Spinal and medullary lamina I projection to nucleus submedius in medial thalamus: A possible pain center. *Journal of Neurophysiology 45*: 443–466, 1981; Peschanski M, and Besson JM. A spino-reticulo-thalamic pathway in the rat: An anatomical study with reference to pain transmission. *Neuroscience 12*(1):165–78, 1984; Vertes RP, Martin GF, and Waltzer R. An autoradiographic analysis of ascending projections from the medullary reticular formation in the rat. *Neuroscience 19*: 873–898, 1986.

In addition to the reticular formation as discussed here, there are other pathways, described primarily in the rodent, that are located in the upper brainstem, receive inputs from exclusively nociceptive spinal cord neurons, and send axons to subcortical limbic structures (amygdala, hypothalamus). The role of these pathways in human pain is unknown but could include affective and autonomic responses to noxious stimulation (Bernard JF, Bester H, and Besson JM. Involvement of the spino-parabrachio-amygdaloid and -hypothalamic pathways in the autonomic and affective emotional aspects of pain. *Progress in Brain Research 107*: 243–255, 1996).

15. Willis WD, and Westlund KN. Neuroanatomy of the pain system and of the pathways that modulate pain. *Journal of Clinical Neurophysiology 14*: 2–31, 1997; Siegel JM. Behavioral functions of the reticular formation. *Brain Research Reviews 1*: 69–105, 1979; Casey KL, and Morrow TJ. Effect of medial bulboreticular and raphe nuclear lesions on the excitation and modulation of supraspinal nocifensive behaviors in the cat. *Brain Research 501*: 150–161, 1989.

16. Rumelhart DE, Hinton GE, and McClelland JL. A general framework for parallel distributed processing. In: Rumelhart DE, and McClelland JL. (Eds.), *Parallel Distributed Processing: Explorations in the Microstructure of Cognition*, Chapter 2. Cambridge, MA: MIT Press, 1986, pp. 45–76.

17. Melzack R, and Casey KL. Sensory, motivational, and central control determinants of pain. In: Kenshalo DR (Ed.), *The Skin Senses*. Springfield, IL: C.C. Thomas, 1968, pp. 423–439. See also: Price DD. Psychological and neural mechanisms of the affective dimension of pain. *Science 288*: 1769–1772, 2000. The latter article decomposes the affective component of pain into an immediate (primary) and a delayed (secondary) unpleasantness that is activated by serial, rather than parallel mechanisms.

18. Kim JS. Patterns of sensory abnormality in cortical stroke: Evidence for a dichotomized sensory system. *Neurology 68*: 174–180, 2007; Semmes J, Porter L, and Randolph MC. Further studies of anterior postcentral lesions in monkeys. *Cortex 10*: 55–68, 1974; Knecht S, Kunesch E, and Schnitzler A. Parallel and serial processing of haptic information in man: Effects of parietal lesions on sensorimotor hand function. *Neuropsychologia 34*: 669–687, 1996.

19. Merskey H, and Bogduk N. *Classification of Chronic Pain: Descriptions of Chronic Pain Syndromes and Definitions of Pain Terms*. Seattle: IASP Press, 1994, p. 222.

20. Melzack R. The McGill Pain Questionnaire: Major properties and scoring methods. *Pain 1*: 277–299, 1975.
    Melzack R. The short-form McGill Pain Questionnaire. *Pain 30*: 191–197, 1987; Price DD, McGrath PA, Rafii A, and Buckingham B. The validation of visual analogue scales as ratio scale measures for chronic and experimental pain. *Pain 17*: 45–56, 1983.

21. Brotis AG, Kapsalaki EZ, Paterakis K, Smith JR, and Fountas KN. Historic evolution of open cingulectomy and stereotactic cingulotomy in the management of medically intractable psychiatric disorders, pain and drug addiction. *Stereotactic and Functional Neurosurgery 87*: 271–291, 2009; Valenstein ES. *Brain Control: A Critical Examination of Brain Stimulation and Psychosurgery*. New York: John Wiley and Sons, Inc., 1973, p. 407.

22. Mendell LM, and Wall PD. Presynaptic hyperpolarization: A role for fine afferent fibres. *Journal of Physiology 172*: 274–294, 1964; Mendell LM. Physiological properties of unmyelinated fiber projection to the spinal cord. *Experimental Neurology 16*: 316–332, 1966. These reports introduced the terms "wide dynamic range" and "windup" to the neurophysiological literature.

23. Willis WD, Trevino DL, Coulter JD, and Maunz RA. Responses of primate spinothalamic tract neurons to natural stimulation of hindlimb. *Journal of Neurophysiology 37*: 358–372, 1974; Chung JM, Kenshalo DR Jr, Gerhart KD, and Willis WD. Excitation of primate

spinothalamic neurons by cutaneous C-fiber volleys. *Journal of Neurophysiology 42*: 1354–1369, 1979; Kenshalo DR Jr, Leonard RB, Chung JM, and Willis WD. Responses of primate spinothalamic neurons to graded and to repeated noxious heat stimulus. *Journal of Neurophysiology 42*: 1370–1389, 1979. The latter two papers reintroduced the term "wide dynamic range" (as WDR) and added "high threshold" (HT) to describe neurons responding only to noxious stimulation. HT later became synonymous with "nociceptive specific" (NS).

24. These articles summarize the arguments against the "labeled line" concept of neuronal coding of pain: Price DD, Greenspan JD, and Dubner R. Neurons involved in the exteroceptive function of pain. *Pain 106*: 215–219, 2003; Green BG. Temperature perception and nociception. *Journal of Neurobiology 61*: 13–29, 2004.

25. Melzack R, and Casey KL. Sensory, motivational, and central control determinants of pain. In: Kenshalo DR (Ed.), *The Skin Senses*. Springfield, IL: C.C. Thomas, 1968, pp. 423–439.

Chapter 5

1. Hebb DO. *The Organization of Behavior*. New York: John Wiley and Sons, 1949; reprint edition, 2002, Lawrence Erlbaum Associates, Mahwah, NJ, p. 335.

2. Ibid. p. 5.

3. Blinkov SM, and Glezer II. *The Human Brain in Figures and Tables*. New York: Basic Books (Plenum Press), 1968 (they estimate only 2000 axons in the STT); Swanson LW. Mapping the human brain: past, present, and future. *Trends in Neurosciences 18*: 471–474, 1995; Cheema SS, Rustioni A, and Whitsel BL. Light and electron microscopic evidence for a direct corticospinal projection to superficial laminae of the dorsal horn in cats and monkeys. *Journal of Comparative Neurology 225*: 276–290, 1984; Ralston DD, and Ralston HJ, III. The terminations of corticospinal tract axons in the macaque monkey. *Journal of Comparative Neurology 242*: 325–337, 1985; Jones EG. Thalamic circuitry and thalamocortical synchrony. *Philosophical Transactions of the Royal Society London B 357*: 1659 1673, 2002.

4. Hagbarth KE, and Fex J. Centrifugal influences on single unit activity in spinal sensory paths. *Journal of Neurophysiology 22*: 321–338, 1959; Hagbarth KE, and Kerr DI. Central influences on spinal afferent conduction. *Journal of Neurophysiology 17*: 295–307, 1954.

5. Poggio GF, and Mountcastle VB. A study of the functional contributions of the lemniscal and spinothalamic systems to somatic sensibility. *Bulletin of Johns Hopkins Hospital 108*: 266–316, 1960; Casey KL. Unit analysis of nociceptive mechanisms in the thalamus of the awake squirrel monkey. *Journal of Neurophysiology 29*: 727–750, 1966; Reynolds D. Surgery in the rat during electrical analgesia induced by focal brain stimulation. *Science 164*: 444–445, 1969. Analgesia was restricted to parts of the body, and some of the effective stimulation sites appeared to be rewarding (supported self-stimulation) (Mayer DJ, Wolfle TL, Akil H, Carder B, and Liebeskind JC. Analgesia from electrical stimulation in the brain of the rat. *Science 174*: 1351–1354, 1971.)

6. Coulter JD, Maunz RA, and Willis WD. Effects of stimulation of sensorimotor cortex on primate spinothalamic tract neurons. *Brain Research 65*: 351–356, 1974; Zhang D, Owens CM, and Willis WD. Two forms of inhibition of spinothalamic tract neurons produced by stimulation of the periaqueductal gray and the cerebral cortex. *Journal of Neurophysiology 65*: 1567–1579, 1991 (and references therein to earlier studies).

7. For a review of this topic, see: Willis WD Jr. Dorsal root potentials and dorsal root reflexes: A double-edged sword. *Experimental Brain Research 124*: 395–421, 1999; Rudomin P. In search of lost presynaptic Inhibition. *Experimental Brain Research 196*: 139–151, 2009.

8. Lloyd DPC, and McIntyre AK. On the origins of dorsal root potentials. *Journal of General Physiology 32*: 409–443, 1949; Wall PD. The origin of a spinal cord slow potential. *Journal of Physiology 164*: 508–526, 1962; Mendell L. Properties and distribution of peripherally evoked presynaptic hyperpolarization in cat lumbar spinal cord. *Journal of Physiology 226*: 769–792, 1972; Marchand S, Charest J, Li J, Chenard JR, Lavignolle B, and Laurencelle L. Is TENS purely a placebo effect? A controlled study on chronic low back pain. *Pain 54*: 99–106, 1993; Sluka KA, and Walsh D. Transcutaneous electrical nerve stimulation: Basic science mechanisms and clinical effectiveness. *Journal of Pain 4*: 109–121, 2003; Dubinsky RM, and Miyasaki J. Assessment: Efficacy of transcutaneous electric nerve stimulation in the treatment of pain in neurologic disorders (an evidence-based review). *Neurology 74*: 173–176, 2010; Mendell LM. Constructing and deconstructing the gate theory of pain. *Pain 155*: 210–216, 2014.

9. Pert CB, and Snyder SH. Opiate receptor: Demonstration in nervous tissue. *Science 179*: 1011–1014, 1973; Hughes J. Isolation of an endogenous compound from the brain with pharmacological properties similar to morphine. *Brain Research 88*: 295–308, 1975; Hughes J, Smith T, Morgan B, and Fothergill L. Purification and properties of encephalin: The possible endogenous ligand for the morphine receptor. *Life Science 16*: 1753–1758, 1975; LaMotte C, Pert CB, and Snyder SH. Opiate receptor binding in primate spinal cord: Distribution and changes after dorsal root section. *Brain Research 112*: 407–412, 1976.

   In the CNS, high concentrations of opiate receptors are found subcortically in the thalamus, hypothalamus, basal ganglia, and reticular formation of the midbrain and brainstem. Opioid receptor binding studies may not distinguish among the several types of opioid receptors in the CNS, such as mu, kappa, and delta, which have different and distinct pharmacological properties. Some other receptor-locating agents bind to receptors for nociceptin, a neurotransmitter that has unique functional properties that contrast with those of the classical analgesic mu opioid agonists (Witta J, Palkovits M, Rosenberger J, and Cox BM. Distribution of nociceptin/orphanin FQ in adult human brain. *Brain Research 997*: 24–29, 2004). There are also important species differences in the distribution of the different types of opioid receptors.

10. Devane WA, Hanus L, Breuer A, Pertwee RG, Stevenson LA, Griffin G, Gibson D, Mandelbaum A, Etinger A, and Mechoulam R. Isolation and structure of a brain constituent that binds to the cannabinoid receptor. *Science 258*: 1946–1949, 1992; Howlett AC, Bidaut-Russell M, Devane WA, Melvin LS, Johnson MR, and Herkenham M. The cannabinoid receptor: Biochemical, anatomical and behavioral characterization. *Trends in Neurosciences 13*: 420–423, 1990.

11. Mogil JS, Simmonds K, and Simmonds MJ. Pain research from 1975 to 2007: A categorical and bibliometric meta-trend analysis of every research paper published in the journal, *Pain. Pain 142*: 48–58, 2009.

Chapter 6

1. Melzack R. The McGill Pain Questionnaire: Major properties and scoring methods. *Pain 1*: 277–299, 1975; Price DD, McGrath PA, Rafii A, and Buckingham B. The validation of visual analogue scales as ratio scale measures for chronic and experimental pain. *Pain 17*: 45–56, 1983.

2. These books provide excellent overviews of the field of psychophysics generally (Gescheider) and as applied to pain research particularly (Price): Gescheider GA.

Psychophysics: The Fundamentals. Mahwah, NJ: Lawrence Erlbaum Associates, 1997, pp. 1–435; Price DD. *Psychological and Neural Mechanisms of Pain.* New York: Raven Press, 1988, pp. 1–241; Price DD. *Psychological Mechanisms of Pain and Analgesia.* Seattle: IASP Press, 1999, pp. 1–248.

3. Taylor DJ, McGillis SLB, and Greenspan JD. Body site variation of heat pain sensitivity. *Somatosensory and Motor Research 10*: 455–465, 1993.

4. Heinbecker P, and Bishop GH. The mechanism of painful sensations. *Proceedings of the Association for Research on Nervous and Mental Disease 15*: 226–238, 1934.

5. Cavanaugh DJ, Lee H, Lo L, Shields SD, Zylka MJ, Basbaum AI, and Anderson DJ. Distinct subsets of unmyelinated primary sensory fibers mediate behavioral responses to noxious thermal and mechanical stimuli. *Proceedings of the National Academy of Sciences USA 106*: 9075–9080, 2009; Shields SD, Cavanaugh DJ, Lee H, Anderson DJ, and Basbaum AI. Pain behavior in the formalin test persists after ablation of the great majority of C-fiber nociceptors. *Pain 151*: 422–429, 2010; Snider WD, and McMahon SB. Tackling pain at the source: New ideas about nociceptors. *Neuron 20*: 629–632, 1998.

6. Adriaensen H, Gybels J, Handwerker HO, and Van Hees J. Response properties of thin myelinated (A-delta) fibers in human skin nerves. *Journal of Neurophysiology 49*: 111–122, 1983; Loken LS, Wessberg J, Morrison I, McGlone F, and Olausson H. Coding of pleasant touch by unmyelinated afferents in humans. *Nature Neuroscience 12*: 1, 2009; Olausson H, Lamarre Y, Backlund H, Morin C, Wallin BG, Starck G, Ekholm S, Strigo I, Worsley K, Vallbo AB, and Bushnell MC. Unmyelinated tactile afferents signal touch and project to insular cortex. *Nature Neuroscience 5*: 900–904, 2002; Vallbo AB, Olausson H, and Wessberg J. Unmyelinated afferents constitute a second system coding tactile stimuli of the human hairy skin. *Journal of Neurophysiology 81*: 2753–2763, 1999.

7. Hagbarth KE, and Vallbo AB. Mechanoreceptor activity recorded percutaneously with semi-microelectrodes in human peripheral nerves. *Acta Physiologica Scandinavica 69*: 121–122, 1967; Vallbo AB, and Hagbarth KE. Activity from skin mechanoreceptors recorded percutaneously in awake human subjects. *Experimental Neurology 21*: 270–289, 1968.

8. Torebjork HE, and Hallin RG. Identification of afferent C units in intact human skin nerves. *Brain Research 67*: 387–403, 1974; Van Hees J, and Gybels JM. Pain related to single afferent C fibers from human skin. *Brain Research 48*: 397–400, 1972.

9. Adriaensen H, Gybels J, Handwerker HO, and Van Hees J. Response properties of thin myelinated (A-delta) fibers in human skin nerves. *Journal of Neurophysiology 49*: 111–122, 1983.

10. Schmidt R, Schmelz M, Forster C, Ringkamp M, Torebjork E, and Handwerker H. Novel classes of responsive and unresponsive C nociceptors in human skin. *Journal of Neuroscience 15*: 333–341, 1995.

11. Heinbecker P, and Bishop GH. The mechanism of painful sensations. *Proceedings of the Association for Research on Nervous and Mental Disease 15*: 226–238, 1934.

12. The inflammatory process is among the most ancient and complex of all biological mechanisms. The literature on inflammation is huge and growing. If you wish to pursue this topic in more depth, the following excellent reviews will lead you deeply into the forest: Henao-Mejia J, Elinav E, Strowig T, and Flavell RA. Inflammasomes: Far beyond inflammation. *Nature Immunology 13*: 321–324, 2012; Lamkanfi M, and Dixit VM. Inflammasomes and their roles in health and disease. *Annual Review of Cell and Developmental Biology 28*: 137–161, 2012; Medzhitov R. Origin and physiological roles of inflammation. *Nature 454*: 428–435, 2008.

13. Schmidt R, Schmelz M, Forster C, Ringkamp M, Torebjork E, and Handwerker H. Novel classes of responsive and unresponsive C nociceptors in human skin. *Journal of Neuroscience 15*: 333–341, 1995.

14. A rather colloquial phrase used liberally even in the most prestigious peer-reviewed scientific journals.

15. Basbaum AI, Bautista DM, Scherrer G, and Julius D. Cellular and molecular mechanisms of pain. *Cell 139*: 267–284, 2009.

16. Ibid. 275–277.

17. Sommer C, Leinders M, and Uceyler N. Inflammation in the pathophysiology of neuropathic pain. *Pain 159*: 595–602, 2018.

18. Trelle S, Reichenbach S, Wandel S, Hildebrand P, Tschannen B, Villiger PM, Egger M, and Juni P. Cardiovascular safety of non-steroidal anti-inflammatory drugs: network meta-analysis. *BMJ 342*: c7086, 2011.

19. Aspirin and related NSAIDs have both peripheral and CNS mechanisms for reducing pain and other symptoms of illness (the "sickness syndrome"). These drugs block the enzymatic conversion of an inflammatory mediator to a molecule a (prostaglandin) that can enter the CNS and activate pain-promoting circuits. See: Saper CB, Romanovsky AA, and Scammell TE. Neural circuitry engaged by prostaglandins during the sickness syndrome. *Nature Neuroscience 15*: 1088–1095, 2012.

20. The action potentials from branches of nociceptive fibers propagate both toward the CNS (called orthodromic conduction) and back along sister branches of that same nerve fiber and into the tissue (called antidromic conduction).

21. Campbell JN, Meyer RA, and LaMotte RH. Sensitization of myelinated nociceptive afferents that innervate monkey hand. *Journal of Neurophysiology 42*: 1669–1679, 1979; LaMotte RH, Thalhammer JG, Torebjork HE, and Robinson CJ. Peripheral neural mechanisms of cutaneous hyperalgesia following mild injury by heat. *Journal of Neuroscience 2*: 765–781, 1982.

Chapter 7

1. Xanthos DN, and Sandkuhler J. Neurogenic neuroinflammation: Inflammatory CNS reactions in response to neuronal activity. *Nature Reviews Neuroscience 15*: 43–53, 2014.

2. Woolf CJ. Evidence for a central component of post-injury pain hypersensitivity. *Nature 306*: 686–688, 1983; Willis WD. Long-term potentiation in spinothalamic neurons. *Brain Research Reviews 40*: 202–214, 2002; Xanthos DN, and Sandkuhler J. Neurogenic neuroinflammation: Inflammatory CNS reactions in response to neuronal activity. *Nature Reviews Neuroscience 15*: 43–53, 2014..

3. The experiences of hyperalgesia (exaggerated pain) and allodynia (pain from normally painless stimulation) can be caused by either PNS or CNS lesions. Allodynia, meaning (from the Greek) "other pain," includes a very unpleasant experience during light brushing; it lacks the distinct sensory quality of normal touch or pain and is sometimes called "dysesthesia" and often characterized as "icky" in colloquial English (see also: Fields HL. Pain: An unpleasant topic. *Pain 6*: S61–S69, 1999). The *causalgia* caused by missile-induced nerve damage is probably mediated by both peripheral and central mechanisms. Surgical interruption of the local autonomic (sympathetic) innervation relieves causalgia in many if not most cases, consistent with a norepinephrine-mediated generation of impulses from damaged sensory nerve fibers. However, it is not clear why these impulses should be painful, suggesting that central sensitization may be necessary also

(see: Livingston WK. *Pain and Suffering*. Seattle: IASP Press, 1998, pp. 103–117; Richards RL. Causalgia: A centennial review. *Archives of Neurology 16*: 339–350, 1967; Wall PD, and Gutnick M. Ongoing activity in peripheral nerves: The physiology and pharmacology of impulses originating from a neuroma. *Experimental Neurology 43*: 580–593, 1974; Blumberg H, and Janig W. Discharge pattern of afferent fibers from a neuroma. *Pain 20*: 335–353, 1984.

4. Nathan PW, Noordenbos W, and Wall PD. Ongoing activity in peripheral nerve: Interactions between electrical stimulation and ongoing activity. *Experimental Neurology 38*: 90–98, 1973.

5. Carr AJ, Robertsson O, Graves S, Price AJ, Arden NK, Judge A, and Beard DJ. Knee replacement. *Lancet 379*: 1331–1340, 2012.

6. Finnerup NB, Attal N, Haroutounian S, McNicol E, Baron R, Dworkin RH, Gilron I, Haanpää M, Hansson P, Jensen TS, Kamerman PR, Lund K, Moore A, Raja SN, Rice ASC, Rowbotham M, Sena E, Siddall P, Smith BH, and Wallace M. Pharmacotherapy for neuropathic pain in adults: A systematic review and meta-analysis. *Lancet Neurology 14*: 162–173, 2015; Stahl SM, Porreca F, Taylor CP, Cheung R, Thorpe AJ, and Clair A. The diverse therapeutic actions of pregabalin: Is a single mechanism responsible for several pharmacological activities? *Trends in Pharmacological Sciences 34*: 332–339, 2013; Taylor CP. Mechanisms of analgesia by gabapentin and pregabalin: Calcium channel [alpha]2-[delta] [Cav[alpha]2-[delta]] ligands. *Pain 142*: 13–16, 2009.

7. Beswick AD, Wylde V, Gooberman-Hill R, Blom A, and Dieppe P. What proportion of patients report long-term pain after total hip or knee replacement for osteoarthritis? A systematic review of prospective studies in unselected patients. *BMJ Open 2*: 2012; Graven-Nielsen T, Wodehouse T, Langford RM, Arendt-Nielsen L, and Kidd BL. Normalization of widespread hyperesthesia and facilitated spatial summation of deep-tissue pain in knee osteoarthritis patients after knee replacement. *Arthritis and Rheumatism 64*: 2907–2916, 2012; Skou ST, Graven-Nielsen T, Rasmussen S, Simonsen OH, Laursen MB, and Arendt-Nielsen L. Widespread sensitization in patients with chronic pain after revision total knee arthroplasty. *Pain 154*: 1588–1594, 2013. See also: Nathan PW, Noordenbos W, and Wall PD. Ongoing activity in peripheral nerve: Interactions between electrical stimulation and ongoing activity. *Experimental Neurology 38*: 90–98, 1973.

8. Gracely RH, Lynch SA, and Bennett GJ. Painful neuropathy: Altered central processing maintained dynamically by peripheral input. *Pain 51*: 175–194, 1992; Haroutounian S, Nikolajsen L, Bendtsen TF, Finnerup NB, Kristensen AD, Hasselstrøm JB, and Jensen TS. Primary afferent input critical for maintaining spontaneous pain in peripheral neuropathy. *Pain 155*: 1272–1279, 2014.

9. Saab CY. Pain-related changes in the brain: Diagnostic and therapeutic potentials. *Trends in Neurosciences 35*: 629–637, 2012; Baron R, Hans G, and Dickenson AH. Peripheral input and its importance for central sensitization. *Annals of Neurology 74*: 630–636, 2013; Denk F, McMahon SB, and Tracey I. Pain vulnerability: A neurobiological perspective. *Nature Neuroscience 17*: 192–200, 2014.

10. Tan LL, Pelzer P, Heinl C, Tang W, Gangadharan V, Flor H, Sprengel R, Kuner T, and Kuner R. A pathway from midcingulate cortex to posterior insula gates nociceptive hypersensitivity. *Nature Neuroscience 20*: 1591–1601, 2017.

11. Mogil JS, Yu L, and Basbaum AI. Pain genes? Natural variation and transgenic mutants. *Annual Review of Neuroscience 23*: 777–811, 2000; Plomin R. The role of inheritance in behavior. *Science 248*: 183–188, 1990.

12. Lacroix-Fralish ML, Ledoux JB, and Mogil JS. The Pain Genes Database: An interactive web browser of pain-related transgenic knockout studies. *Pain 131*: 3.e1–4, 2007; Perkins JR, Lees J, Antunes-Martins A, Diboun I, McMahon SB, Bennett DLH, and Orengo C. PainNetworks: A web-based resource for the visualisation of pain-related genes in the context of their network associations. *Pain 154*: 2586.e2581–2586.e2512, 2013.

13. https://www.ncbi.nlm.nih.gov/pmc/articles/PMC4889822/. The functional numerical disparity may be greater because some genes do not encode for proteins. The actual number of proteins is difficult to determine because slight changes in amino acid composition and structural configuration may determine how the molecule functions or is recognized. An estimated range of the total number of unique protein molecules in a typical human cell is generally between 250,000 and about 1,000,000. There are probably many more unique proteins distributed among the many different types of cells, so an estimate of 2,000,000 unique proteins is sometimes given.

14. Waxman SG. Nav1.7, its mutations, and the syndromes that they cause. *Neurology 69*: 505–507, 2007.

15. Lee J-H, Park C-K, Chen G, Han Q, Xie R-G, Liu T, Ji R-R, and Lee S-Y. A monoclonal antibody that targets a NaV1.7 channel voltage sensor for pain and itch relief. *Cell 157*: 1393–1404, 2014.

16. Raouf R, Quick K, and Wood JN. Pain as a channelopathy. *Journal of Clinical Investigation 120*: 3745–3752, 2010.

17. Critchley M. Congenital indifference to pain. *Annals of Internal Medicine 45*: 737–747, 1956; Magee KR, Schneider SF, and Rosenzweig N. Congenital indifference to pain. *Journal of Nervous and Mental Disease 132*: 249–259, 1961; Magee KR. Congenital indifference to pain. *Archives of Neurology 9*: 635–640, 1963; Nagasako EM, Oaklander AL, and Dworkin RH. Congenital insensitivity to pain: An update. *Pain 101*: 213–219, 2003; Cox JJ, Reimann F, Nicholas AK, Thornton G, Roberts E, Springell K, Karbani G, Jafri H, Mannan J, Raashid Y, Al Gazali L, Hamamy H, Valente EM, Gorman S, Williams R, McHale DP, Wood JN, Gribble FM, and Woods CG. An SCN9A channelopathy causes congenital inability to experience pain. *Nature 444*: 894–898, 2006; Swanson AG, Buchan GC, and Alvord EC Jr. Anatomic changes in congenital insensitivity to pain. *Archives of Neurology 12*: 12–18, 1965.

18. Zorina-Lichtenwalter K, Parisien M, and Diatchenko L. Genetic studies of human neuropathic pain conditions: A review. *Pain 159*: 583–594, 2018. See discussion of neuropathic pain in Chapter 9.

19. For a review related to this topic, see: Denk F, McMahon SB, and Tracey I. Pain vulnerability: A neurobiological perspective. *Nature Neuroscience 17*: 192–200, 2014.

Chapter 8

1. Beecher HK. Relationship of significance of wound to pain experienced. *Journal of the American Medical Association 161*: 1609–1613, 1956; Beecher HK. The measurement of pain: Prototype for the quantitative study of subjective responses. *Pharmacological Reviews 9*: 59–209, 1957.

2. Hagbarth KE, and Kerr DI. Central influences on spinal afferent conduction. *Journal of Neurophysiology 17*: 295–307, 1954.; Hagbarth KE, and Fex J. Centrifugal influences on single unit activity in spinal sensory paths. *Journal of Neurophysiology 22*: 321–338, 1959; Casey KL. Unit analysis of nociceptive mechanisms in the thalamus of the awake squirrel monkey. *Journal of Neurophysiology 29*: 727–750, 1966; ; Reynolds D. Surgery in the rat

during electrical analgesia induced by focal brain stimulation. *Science 164*: 444–445, 1969; (Mayer DJ, Wolfle TL, Akil H, Carder B, and Liebeskind JC. Analgesia from electrical stimulation in the brain of the rat. *Science 174*: 1351–1354, 1971.

3. Hoffman DS, Dubner R, Hayes RL, and Medlin TP. Neuronal activity in medullary dorsal horn of awake monkeys trained in a thermal discrimination task. I. Responses to innocuous and noxious thermal stimuli. *Journal of Neurophysiology 46*: 409–427, 1981; Hayes RL, Dubner R, and Hoffman DS. Neuronal activity in medullary dorsal horn of awake monkeys trained in a thermal discrimination task. II. Behavioral modulation of responses to thermal and mechanical stimuli. *Journal of Neurophysiology 46*: 428–443, 1981; Dubner R, Hoffman DS, and Hayes RL. Neuronal activity in medullary dorsal horn of awake monkeys trained in a thermal discrimination task. III. Task-related responses and their functional role. *Journal of Neurophysiology 46*: 444–464, 1981.

4. The following papers review the development of this research area during and for the two decades following the discovery of analgesia evoked by brainstem stimulation: Liebeskind JC, and Paul LA. Psychological and physiological mechanisms of pain. *Annual Review of Psychology 28*: 41–60, 1977; Basbaum AI, and Fields HL. Endogenous pain control systems: Brainstem spinal pathways and endorphin circuitry. *Annual Review of Neuroscience 7*: 309–338, 1984; Fields HL, Heinricher MM, and Mason P. Neurotransmitters in nociceptive modulatory circuits. *Annual Review of Neuroscience 14*: 219–245, 1991.

5. Behbehani MM. Functional characteristics of the midbrain periaqueductal gray. *Progress in Neurobiology 46*: 575–605, 1995; Linnman C, Moulton EA, Barmettler G, Becerra L, and Borsook D. Neuroimaging of the periaqueductal gray: State of the field. *NeuroImage 60*: 505–522, 2012.

6. Melzack R, Stotler WA, and Livingston WK. Effects of discrete brain stem lesions in cats on perception of noxious stimulation. *Journal of Neurophysiology 21*: 353–367, 1958.

7. Fields HL, Heinricher MM, and Mason P. Neurotransmitters in nociceptive modulatory circuits. *Annual Review of Neuroscience 14*: 219–245, 1991.

8. Bouhassira D, Le Bars D, Bolgert F, Laplane D, and Willer JC. Diffuse noxious inhibitory controls in humans: A neurophysiological investigation of a patient with a form of Brown-Sequard syndrome. *Annals of Neurology 34*: 536–543, 1993. See also: Le Bars D. The whole body receptive field of dorsal horn multireceptive neurones. *Brain Research Reviews 40*: 29–44, 2002; Le Bars D, Dickenson AH, and Besson JM. Diffuse noxious inhibitory controls (DNIC). I. Effects on dorsal horn convergent neurones in the rat. *Pain 6*: 283–304, 1979; Le Bars D, Dickenson AH, and Besson JM. Diffuse noxious inhibitory controls (DNIC). II. Lack of effect on non-convergent neurones, supraspinal involvement and theoretical implications. *Pain 6*: 305–327, 1979.

9. Le Bars D. The whole body receptive field of dorsal horn multireceptive neurones. *Brain Research Reviews 40*: 29–44, 2002.

10. See the following for evidence and discussion about some of these caveats: Holstege JC, and Kuypers HGJM. Brainstem projections to spinal motoneurons: An update. *Neuroscience 23*: 809–822, 1987; Fields HL, Malick A, and Burstein R. Dorsal horn projection targets of ON and OFF cells in the rostral ventromedial medulla. *Journal of Neurophysiology 74*: 1742–1759, 1995; Porreca F, Ossipov MH, and Gebhart GF. Chronic pain and medullary descending facilitation. *Trends in Neurosciences 25*: 319–325, 2002; Ossipov MH, Dussor GO, and Porreca F. Central modulation of pain. *Journal of Clinical Investigation 120*: 3779–3787, 2010; Mason P. Contributions of the medullary raphe and ventromedial reticular region to pain modulation and other homeostatic functions. *Annual Review of Neuroscience 24*: 737–777, 2001; Mason P. Deconstructing endogenous pain modulations.

Journal of Neurophysiology 94: 1659–1663, 2005; Mason P. Medullary circuits for no-ciceptive modulation. *Current Opinion in Neurobiology 22*: 640–645, 2012; Mason P. Ventromedial medulla: pain modulation and beyond. *Journal of Comparative Neurology 493*: 2–8, 2005.

11. Tan LL, Pelzer P, Heinl C, Tang W, Gangadharan V, Flor H, Sprengel R, Kuner T, and Kuner R. A pathway from midcingulate cortex to posterior insula gates nociceptive hyper-sensitivity. *Nature Neuroscience 20*: 1591–1601, 2017.

12. Mehler WR, Feferman ME, and Nauta WJH. Ascending axon degeneration following an-terolateral cordotomy: An experimental study in the monkey. *Brain 83*: 718–750, 1960.

13. For a review of the history and current status of DBS generally, see: Bittar RG, Kar-Purkayastha I, Owen SL, Bear RE, Green A, Wang S, and Aziz TZ. Deep brain stimulation for pain relief: A meta-analysis. *Journal of Clinical Neuroscience 12*: 515–519, 2005; Gybels J, and Kupers R. Deep brain stimulation in the treatment of chronic pain in man: Where and why? *Neurophysiologie Clinique 20*: 389–398, 1990; Iacono RP, and Nashold BS Jr. Mental and behavioral effects of brain stem and hypothalamic stimulation in man. *Human Neurobiology 1*: 273–279, 1982; Kumar K, Toth C, and Nath RK. Deep brain stim-ulation for intractable pain: A 15-year experience. *Neurosurgery 40*: 736–746; discussion 746–737, 1997; Pereira EA, and Aziz TZ. Neuropathic pain and deep brain stimulation. *Neurotherapeutics 11*: 496–507, 2014; Rasche D, Rinaldi PC, Young RF, and Tronnier VM. Deep brain stimulation for the treatment of various chronic pain syndromes. *Neurosurgical Focus 21*: E8, 2006; Richardson DE, and Akil H. Long term results of periventricular gray self-stimulation. *Neurosurgery 1*: 199–202, 1977.

14. Peyron R, Faillenot I, Mertens P, Laurent B, and Garcia-Larrea L. Motor cortex stimulation in neuropathic pain: Correlations between analgesic effect and hemodynamic changes in the brain. A PET study. *NeuroImage 34*: 310–321, 2007; Garcia-Larrea L, and Peyron R. Motor cortex stimulation for neuropathic pain: From phenomenology to mechanisms. *NeuroImage 37* Suppl 1: S71–S79, 2007; Hosomi K, Shimokawa T, Ikoma K, Nakamura Y, Sugiyama K, Ugawa Y, Uozumi T, Yamamoto T, and Saitoh Y. Daily repetitive transcranial magnetic stimulation of primary motor cortex for neuropathic pain: A randomized, multicenter, double-blind, crossover, sham-controlled trial. *Pain 154*: 1065–1072, 2013; Lima MC, and Fregni F. Motor cortex stimulation for chronic pain: Systematic review and meta-analysis of the literature. *Neurology 70*: 2329–2337, 2008; Nuti C, Peyron R, Garcia-Larrea L, Brunon J, Laurent B, Sindou M, and Mertens P. Motor cortex stimula-tion for refractory neuropathic pain: Four year outcome and predictors of efficacy. *Pain 118*: 43–52, 2005; Tsubokawa T, Katayama Y, Yamamoto T, Hirayama T, and Koyama S. Chronic motor cortex stimulation in patients with thalamic pain. *Journal of Neurosurgery 78*: 393–401, 1993.

15. Feedback mechanisms for controlling sensory and motor function are found throughout the CNS. A simple example is the pupillary light reflex. The purpose of the pupillary opening is to expose the retina to light; but too much light can impair vision or even damage the retina. A feedback control mechanism protects the retina. In dimness or dark, the pupil dilates; with light, it constricts. The neural circuits controlling this reflex extend from the retina to the upper brainstem, near the PAG. However, pupil diameter is also affected by brain circuits that participate in cognition, attention, and the elaboration of emotions. For example, pupils dilate during fear, even in a lighted environment.

16. Lenz FA, Seike M, Richardson RT, Lin YC, Baker FH, Khoja I, Jaeger CJ, and Gracely RH. Thermal and pain sensations evoked by microstimulation in the area of human ventrocaudal nucleus. *Journal of Neurophysiology 70*: 200–212, 1993; Weigel R, and Krauss

JK. Center median-parafascicular complex and pain control: Review from a neurosurgical perspective. *Stereotactic and Functional Neurosurgery 82*: 115–126, 2004; Mayer DJ, Price DD, and Becker DP. Neurophysiological characterization of the anterolateral spinal cord neurons contributing to pain perception in man. *Pain 1*: 51–58, 1975; Mazzola L, Isnard J, Peyron R, and Mauguiere F. Stimulation of the human cortex and the experience of pain: Wilder Penfield's observations revisited. *Brain 135*: 631–640, 2012; Nair DR, Najm I, Bulacio J, and Luders H. Painful auras in focal epilepsy. *Neurology 57*: 700–702, 2001; Isnard J, Magnin M, Jung J, Mauguişre F, and Garcia-Larrea L. Does the insula tell our brain that we are in pain? *Pain 152*: 946–951, 2011.

17. Vierck CJ, Whitsel BL, Favorov OV, Brown AW, and Tommerdahl M. Role of primary somatosensory cortex in the coding of pain. *Pain 154*: 334–344, 2013.

18. Schmahmann JD, and Leifer D. Parietal pseudothalamic pain syndrome: Clinical features and anatomic correlates. *Archives of Neurology 49*: 1032–1037, 1992; Bowsher D. Central pain: Clinical and physiological characteristics. *Journal of Neurology, Neurosurgery, and Psychiatry 61*: 62–69, 1996; Bowsher D, Leijon G, and Thuomas KA. Central poststroke pain: Correlation of MRI with clinical pain characteristics and sensory abnormalities. *Neurology 51*: 1352–1358, 1998; Boivie J. Central post-stoke pain. Ch.48 In: Cervero F, and Jensen TS (Eds.), *Pain, Handbook of Neurology*, Volume 81, Chapter 48. Edinburgh: Elsevier, 2006, pp. 715–730.

19. Bromm B, and Lorenz J. Neurophysiological evaluation of pain. *Electroencephalography and Clinical Neurophysiology 107*: 227–253, 1998; Hu L, Cai MM, Xiao P, Luo F, and Iannetti GD. Human brain responses to concomitant stimulation of Adelta and C nociceptors. *Journal of Neuroscience 34*: 11439–11451, 2014; Lorenz J, and Garcia-Larrea L. Contribution of attentional and cognitive factors to laser-evoked brain potentials. *Clinical Neurophysiology 33*: 293–301, 2003; Ploner M, Schmitz F, Freund HJ, and Schnitzler A. Parallel activation of primary and secondary somatosensory cortices in human pain processing. *Journal of Neurophysiology 81*: 3100–3104, 1999; Schnitzler A, and Ploner M. Neurophysiology and functional neuroanatomy of pain perception. *Journal of Clinical Neurophysiology 17*: 592–603, 2000; Wager TD, Matre D, and Casey KL. Placebo effects in laser-evoked pain potentials. *Brain, Behavior, and Immunity 20*: 219–230, 2006; Tiemann L, May ES, Postorino M, Schulz E, Nickel MM, Bingel U, and Ploner M. Differential neurophysiological correlates of bottom-up and top-down modulations of pain. *Pain 156*: 289–296, 2015.

20. Buzśaki G, and Wang XJ. Mechanisms of gamma oscillations. *Annual Review of Neuroscience 35*: 203–225, 2012; Gross J, Schnitzler A, Timmermann L, and Ploner M. Gamma oscillations in human primary somatosensory cortex reflect pain perception. *PloS Biology 5*: e133, 2007.

21. For a thorough discussion of neuropathic pain due to disease or trauma affecting the PNS or CNS, see: Campbell JN, and Meyer RA. Mechanisms of neuropathic pain. *Neuron 52*: 77–92, 2006; Boivie J. Central pain. In: Wall PD, and Melzack R. (Eds.), *Textbook of Pain*, Edinburgh: Churchill-Livingstone, 1994.

Chapter 9

1. In radiology, tomography is a technique for focusing multiple x-ray exposures on an area of interest within a plane of view.

2. Oldendorf WH. The quest for an image of brain: A brief historical and technical review of brain imaging techniques. *Neurology 28*: 517–33, 1978; Hounsfield GN. Computed

medical imaging. Nobel lecture, December 8, 1979. *Journal of Computer Assisted Tomography* 4: 665–674, 1980.

3. Bogousslavsky J, Regli F, and Uske A. Thalamic infarcts: Clinical syndromes, etiology, and prognosis. *Neurology 38*: 837–848, 1988; Fisher CM. Lacunar strokes and infarcts: A review. *Neurology 32*: 871–876, 1982; Davison C, and Schick W. Spontaneous pain and other subjective sensory disturbances. *AMA Archives of Neurology and Psychiatry 34*: 1204–1237, 1935; Schmahmann JD. Vascular syndromes of the thalamus. *Stroke 34*: 2264–2278, 2003; Schmahmann JD, and Leifer D. Parietal pseudothalamic pain syndrome: Clinical features and anatomic correlates. *Archives of Neurology 49*: 1032–1037, 1992; Cohen RA, Kaplan RF, Moser DJ, Jenkins MA, and Wilkinson H. Impairments of attention after cingulotomy. *Neurology 53*: 819–824, 1999.

4. The term "magnetic resonance" refers to the electromagnetic signal produced by the rhythmic reorientation of the nuclei of hydrogen atoms (protons) that have had their oscillations temporarily displaced by electromagnetic pulses applied repetitively to tissue within a magnetic field. "Imaging" refers to the detection and spatial localization of this signal. The strength of the proton signal is different among areas dominated by cell bodies (gray matter), areas containing many myelinated axons (white matter), and cerebrospinal fluid, thus revealing internal brain structure.

5. Bassetti C, Bogousslavsky J, Mattle H, and Bernasconi A. Medial medullary stroke: Report of seven patients and review of the literature. *Neurology 48*: 882–890, 1997; Bassetti C, Bogousslavsky J, and Regli F. Sensory syndromes in parietal stroke. *Neurology 43*: 1942–1949, 1993; Greenspan JD, Lee RR, and Lenz FA. Pain sensitivity alterations as a function of lesion location in the parasylvian cortex. *Pain 81*: 273–282, 1999; Kim JH, Greenspan JD, Coghill RC, Ohara S, and Lenz FA. Lesions limited to the human thalamic principal somatosensory nucleus (ventral caudal) are associated with loss of cold sensations and central pain. *Journal of Neuroscience 27*: 4995–5004, 2007; Cereda C, Ghika J, Maeder P, and Bogousslavsky J. Strokes restricted to the insular cortex. *Neurology 59*: 1950–1955, 2002; Bowsher D, Leijon G, and Thuomas KA. Central poststroke pain: Correlation of MRI with clinical pain characteristics and sensory abnormalities. *Neurology 51*: 1352–1358, 1998.

6. Ploner M, Freund HJ, and Schnitzler A. Pain affect without pain sensation in a patient with a postcentral lesion. *Pain 81*: 211–214, 1999. I have seen a few similar cases in practice but could not document the findings adequately.

7. Some have objected to the use of "parallel" to describe the relationship between the affective and discriminative (pure sensory) components of pain (see: Price DD. Psychological and neural mechanisms of the affective dimension of pain. *Science 288*: 1769–1772, 2000; Price DD. *Psychological Mechanisms of Pain and Analgesia*. Seattle: IASP Press, 1999, pp. 248.). The objections seem to be based on anatomy and timing. *Anatomically*, the most direct and secure connections within the circuits that mediate these two dimensions are certainly separate and can be regarded as parallel in that sense; however, they also have less direct and secure connections with one another so that nociceptive neurons may be found (in differing proportions) in both circuits. Pure CNS parallelism is rare, if it exists at all. The *temporal* objection is that some early stage or low level of nociceptive detection is accompanied by only "rudimentary" negative affect or "immediate pain unpleasantness" (Price, 2000). The author refers to the brief noxious heat used in his laboratory experiments as "not unpleasant" (*sic*; Price, 1999, p. 6) to normal persons. Accordingly, the seriously (presumably nonrudimentary) affective component of pain ("secondary unpleasantness") must follow this initial (rudimentarily affective?) nociceptive detection in a serial, not a parallel, process. This distinction raises an interesting question of mechanistic detail, but

whether activated in purely parallel or partially serial form, there is no doubt that the pains of everyday life and in the clinic are intrinsically unpleasant and require the conjoint participation of interacting but anatomically and physiologically distinct neural circuits. See also Chapter 4, section on "Pain: A Synthetic Experience and a New Conceptual Model", and Chapter 10, section on "Pain Emerges from the Conjoint Activation of Structures Mediating Sensory, Affective, and Cognitive Functions."

8. Ebner TJ, and Chen G. Use of voltage-sensitive dyes and optical recordings in the central nervous system. *Progress in Neurobiology 46*: 463–506, 1995; Peterka DS, Takahashi H, and Yuste R. Imaging voltage in neurons. *Neuron 69*: 9–21, 2011.

9. MRS is a method for detecting the presence and relative (to another "baseline" chemical such as creatine) amount of a specific chemical, in this case within an anatomically specified volume of the brain. The physical principle behind MRS is similar to that of MRI except that the target compound (compound of interest) emits an electromagnetic signal at a specific frequency, the amplitude of which must be extracted in the analysis. See: Duncan JS. Magnetic resonance spectroscopy. *Epilepsia 37*: 598–605, 1996; Rae CD. A guide to the metabolic pathways and function of metabolites observed in human brain 1H magnetic resonance spectra. *Neurochemical Research 39*: 1–36, 2014.

10. Roy CS, and Sherrington CS. On the regulation of the blood-supply of the brain. *Journal of Physiology (London) 11*: 85–108, 1890.

11. In reviewing the history linking cerebral blood flow to neuronal activity, Raichle cites a 1928 report in which the sound of increased turbulent blood flow through a vascular malformation in a patient's visual cortex could be heard through a stethoscope, and by the patient, when the patient is engaged in reading (Raichle ME. Behind the scenes of functional brain imaging: A historical and physiological perspective. *Proceeding of the National Academy of Sciences USA 95*: 765–772, 1998.)

12. Haydon PG, and Carmignoto G. Astrocyte control of synaptic transmission and neurovascular coupling. *Physiological Review 86*: 1009–1031, 2006.

13. There is much discussion about this in the literature, but it has little to do with understanding how well increased rCBF serves as a surrogate measure of neuronal activity. A short explanation is that the excess of blood oxygen and glucose may be more apparent than real because the oxygen demand is relatively low while the metabolic (glucose) demands of glial cells is high during the neuronal release and recycling of neurotransmitter. The overshoot, therefore, may supply excessive oxygen but just the right amount of glucose for nonoxidative glucose metabolism (anaerobic glycolysis) by astrocytes. See: Raichle ME. Neuroscience: The brain's dark energy. *Science 314*: 1249–1250, 2006; Raichle ME, and Mintun MA. Brain work and brain imaging. *Annual Review of Neuroscience 29*: 449–476, 2006.

14. It has been possible to estimate that, from the ~18,000 neurons in each cortical column, approximately 4500 action potentials are generated during 100 milliseconds following a single 200-millisecond displacement of a rat's whisker. (Most neurons generated less than one action potential per stimulus.) In the optical imaging experiment described earlier, five similar stimuli were delivered over the 1-second stimulation period. Therefore, that hemodynamic response roughly estimates the generation of 22,500 action potentials from a single cortical column within an area about 167 times larger than the area of the active column. de Kock CP, Bruno RM, Spors H, and Sakmann B. Layer- and cell-type-specific suprathreshold stimulus representation in

rat primary somatosensory cortex. *Journal of Physiology 581*: 139–154, 2007; Meyer HS, Wimmer VC, Oberlaender M, de Kock CPJ, Sakmann B, and Helmstaedter M. Number and laminar distribution of neurons in a thalamocortical projection column of rat vibrissal cortex. *Cerebral Cortex 20*: 2277–2286, 2010; Devor A, Dunn AK, Andermann ML, Ulbert I, Boas DA, and Dale AM. Coupling of total hemoglobin concentration, oxygenation, and neural activity in rat somatosensory cortex. *Neuron 39*: 353–359, 2003; Devor A, Ulbert I, Dunn AK, Narayanan SN, Jones SR, Andermann ML, Boas DA, and Dale AM. Coupling of the cortical hemodynamic response to cortical and thalamic neuronal activity. *Proceedings of the National Academy of Sciences USA 102*: 3822–3827, 2005.

15. Mathiesen C, Caesar K, Akgoren N, and Lauritzen M. Modification of activity-dependent increases of cerebral blood flow by excitatory synaptic activity and spikes in rat cerebellar cortex. *Journal of Physiology 512*: 555–566, 1998; Thomsen K, Offenhauser N, and Lauritzen M. Principal neuron spiking: Neither necessary nor sufficient for cerebral blood flow in rat cerebellum. *Journal of Physiology 560*: 181–189, 2004.

16. A full presentation of the physics of fMRI is available in: Buxton RB. *Introduction to Functional Magnetic Resonance Imaging*. Cambridge, UK: Cambridge University Press, 2002, pp. 523.

17. Logothetis NK. What we can do and what we cannot do with fMRI. *Nature 453*: 869–878, 2008; Aguirre GK. Functional neuroimaging: Technical, logical, and social perspectives. *Hastings Center Report 45*: S8–S18, 2014. See also: https://cfn.upenn.edu/aguirre/wiki/public:neurons_in_a_voxel.

18. Gronenberg W. Structure and function of ant (Hymenoptera: Formicidae) brains: Strength in numbers. *Myrmecological News 11*: 25–36, 2008; Strausfeld NJ. *Atlas of an Insect Brain*. Berlin: Springer-Verlag, 1976, p. 211, pp. 49–50; Strausfeld NJ, Hansen L, Li Y, Gomez RS, and Ito K. Evolution, discovery, and interpretations of arthropod mushroom bodies. *Learning and Memory 5*: 11–37, 1998.

19. Friston KJ, Frith CD, Liddle PF, and Frackowiak RS. Comparing functional (PET) images: The assessment of significant change. *Journal of Cerebral Blood Flow and Metabolism 11*: 690–699, 1991; Friston KJ, Holmes A, Poline JB, Price CJ, and Frith CD. Detecting activations in PET and fMRI: Levels of inference and power. *NeuroImage 4*: 223–235, 1996.

20. Reivich M, Kuhl D, Wolf A, Greenberg J, Phelps M, Ido T, Casella V, Fowler J, Hoffman E, Alavi A, Som P, and Sokoloff L. The [18F]fluorodeoxyglucose method for the measurement of local cerebral glucose utilization in man. *Circulation Research 44*: 127–137, 1979; Phelps ME, Kuhl DE, and Mazziota JC. Metabolic mapping of the brain's response to visual stimulation: Studies in humans. *Science 211*: 1445–1448, 1981.

21. Fox PT, Mintun MA, Raichle ME, and Herscovitch P. A noninvasive approach to quantitative functional brain mapping with H2 (15)O and positron emission tomography. *Journal of Cerebral Blood Flow and Metabolism 4*: 329–333, 1984.

22. Buxton RB. *Introduction to Functional Magnetic Resonance Imaging*. Cambridge, UK: Cambridge University Press, 2002, Chapter 15.

23. Heiss WD, and Herholz K. Brain receptor imaging. *Journal of Nuclear Medicine 47*: 302–312, 2006.

24. Ashurner J, and Friston KJ. Voxel-based morphometry: The methods. *NeuroImage 11*: 805–821, 2000.

Chapter 10

1. Jensen KB, Regenbogen C, Ohse MC, Frasnelli J, Freiherr J, and Lundstrom JN. Brain activations during pain: A neuroimaging meta-analysis of patients with pain and healthy controls. *Pain 157*: 1279–1286, 2016.

2. Gusnard DA, Raichle ME, and Raichle ME. Searching for a baseline: Functional imaging and the resting human brain. *Nature Reviews Neuroscience 2*: 685–694, 2001; Raichle ME, MacLeod AM, Snyder AZ, Powers WJ, Gusnard DA, and Shulman GL. A default mode of brain function. *Proceedings of the National Academy of Science USA 98*: 676–682, 2001; Shulman RG, Rothman DL, Behar KL, and Hyder F. Energetic basis of brain activity: Implications for neuroimaging. *Trends in Neurosciences 27*: 489–495, 2004.

3. Madsen PL, Holm S, Herning M, and Lassen NA. Average blood flow and oxygen uptake in the human brain during resting wakefulness: A critical appraisal of the Kety-Schmidt technique. *Journal of Cerebral Blood Flow and Metabolism 13*: 646–655, 1993.

4. Nathan PW, Noordenbos W, and Wall PD. Ongoing activity in peripheral nerve: Interactions between electrical stimulation and ongoing activity. *Experimental Neurology 38*: 90–98, 1973.

5. Simpson JR Jr, Drevets WC, Snyder AZ, Gusnard DA, and Raichle ME. Emotion-induced changes in human medial prefrontal cortex: II. During anticipatory anxiety. *Proceedings of the National Academy of Science USA 98*: 688–693, 2001; Simpson JR Jr, Snyder AZ, Gusnard DA, and Raichle ME. Emotion-induced changes in human medial prefrontal cortex: I. During cognitive task performance. *Proceedings of the National Academy of Science USA 98*: 683–687, 2001.

6. Papez JW. A proposed mechanism of emotion. *Archives of Neurological Psychiatry 38*: 725–743, 1937; MacLean PD. Psychosomatic disease and the "visceral brain." *Psychosomatic Medicine 11*: 338–353, 1949.

7. Damasio AR, Grabowski TJ, Bechara A, Damasio H, Ponto LL, Parvizi J, and Hichwa RD. Subcortical and cortical brain activity during the feeling of self-generated emotions. *Nature Neuroscience 3*: 1049–1056, 2000.

8. Talbot JD, Marrett S, Evans AC, Meyer E, Bushnell MC, and Duncan GH. Multiple representations of pain in human cerebral cortex. *Science 251*: 1355–1358, 1991; Jones AK, Brown WD, Friston KJ, Qi LY, and Frackowiak RS. Cortical and subcortical localization of response to pain in man using positron emission tomography. *Proceedings of the Royal Society London [Biology] 244*: 39–44, 1991; Casey KL, Minoshima S, Berger KL, Koeppe RA, Morrow TJ, and Frey KA. Positron emission tomographic analysis of cerebral structures activated specifically by repetitive noxious heat stimuli. *Journal of Neurophysiology 71*: 802–807, 1994; Coghill RC, Talbot JD, Evans AC, Meyer E, Gjedde A, Bushnell MC, and Duncan GH. Distributed processing of pain and vibration by the human brain. *Journal of Neuroscience 14*: 4095–4108, 1994.

9. Rainville P, Duncan GH, Price DD, Carrier M, and Bushnell MC. Pain affect encoded in human anterior cingulate but not somatosensory cortex. *Science 277*: 968–971, 1997. In the case of hypnosis, it is apparently possible to have painless nociception, recalling the issue of parallel vs. serial pain processing discussed previously.

10. Lorenz J, Cross D, Minoshima S, Morrow T, Paulson P, and Casey K. A unique representation of heat allodynia in the human brain. *Neuron 35*: 383–393, 2002.

11. Ploner M, Gross J, Timmermann L, and Schnitzler A. Cortical representation of first and second pain sensation in humans. *Proceedings of the National Academy of Science USA 99*: 12444–12448, 2002. See also: Ploner M, Freund HJ, and Schnitzler A. Pain affect

without pain sensation in a patient with a postcentral lesion. *Pain 81*: 211–214, 1999.; Bastuji H, Frot M, Perchet C, Magnin M, and Garcia-Larrea L. Pain networks from the inside: Spatiotemporal analysis of brain responses leading from nociception to conscious perception. *Human Brain Mapping* (e-publication 9 July 2016).

12. Ingvar M. Pain and functional imaging. *Philosophical Transactions of the Royal Society of London B:Biological Sciences 354*: 1347–1358, 1999; Peyron R, Laurent B, and Garcia-Larrea L. Functional imaging of brain responses to pain: A review and meta-analysis. *Clinical Neurophysiology 30*: 263–288, 2000; Apkarian AV, Bushnell MC, Treede RD, and Zubieta JK. Human brain mechanisms of pain perception and regulation in health and disease. *European Journal of Pain 9*: 463–484, 2005; Tracey I, and Mantyh PW. The cerebral signature for pain perception and its modulation. *Neuron 55*: 377–391, 2007; Jensen KB, Regenbogen C, Ohse MC, Frasnelli J, Freiherr J, and Lundstrom JN. Brain activations during pain: A neuroimaging meta-analysis of patients with pain and healthy controls. *Pain 157*: 1279–1286, 2016.

13. Bingel U, Quante M, Knab R, Bromm B, Weiller C, and Buchel C. Single trial fMRI reveals significant contralateral bias in responses to laser pain within thalamus and somatosensory cortices. *NeuroImage 18*: 740–748, 2003; Wager TD, Atlas LY, Lindquist MA, Roy M, Woo CW, and Kross E. An fMRI-based neurologic signature of physical pain. *New England Journal of Medicine 368*: 1388–1397, 2013.

14. Melzack R, and Casey KL. Sensory, motivational, and central control determinants of pain. In: Kenshalo DR (Ed.), *The Skin Senses.* Springfield, IL: C.C. Thomas, 1968, pp. 423–439; Merskey H, and Bogduk N. *Classification of Chronic Pain: Descriptions of Chronic Pain Syndromes and Definitions of Pain Terms.* Seattle: IASP Press, 1994, pp. 222.

15. Wager TD, Atlas LY, Lindquist MA, Roy M, Woo CW, and Kross E. An fMRI-based neurologic signature of physical pain. *New England Journal of Medicine 368*: 1388–1397, 2013.

16. Legrain V, Iannetti GD, Plaghki L, and Mouraux A. The pain matrix reloaded: A salience detection system for the body. *Progress in Neurobiology 93*: 111–124, 2011; Mouraux A, Diukova A, Lee MC, Wise RG, and Iannetti GD. A multisensory investigation of the functional significance of the "pain matrix." *NeuroImage 54*: 2237–2249, 2011; Liang M, Mouraux A, and Iannetti GD. Bypassing primary sensory cortices: A direct thalamocortical pathway for transmitting salient sensory information. *Cerebral Cortex 23*: 1–11, 2013.

17. Rauch SL, Savage CR, Alpert NM, Miguel EC, Baer L, Breiter HC, Fischman AJ, Manzo PA, Moretti C, and Jenike MA. A positron emission tomographic study of simple phobic symptom provocation. *Archives of General Psychiatry 52*: 20–28, 1995; Straube T, Mentzel HJ, and Miltner WH. Waiting for spiders: Brain activation during anticipatory anxiety in spider phobics. *NeuroImage 37*: 1427–1436, 2007; Ipser JC, Singh L, and Stein DJ. Meta-analysis of functional brain imaging in specific phobia. *Psychiatry and Clinical Neurosciences 67*: 311–322, 2013.

18. In fact, the putative pain circuitry (sometimes called "pain matrix") is activated by noxious stimuli that are perceived as painful by normal individuals but painless in individuals with congenital insensitivity to pain. See: Salomons TV, Iannetti G, Liang M, and Wood JN. The "pain matrix" in pain-free individuals. *JAMA Neurology 73*: 755–766, 2016. See also the figure and editorial comment in this article: Geha P, and Waxman SG. Pain perception: Multiple matrices or one? *JAMA Neurology 73*: 628–630, 2016.

19. Yarkoni T, Poldrack RA, Nichols TE, Van Essen DC, and Wager TD. Large-scale automated synthesis of human functional neuroimaging data. *Nature Methods 8*: 665–670, 2011.

20. Derbyshire SW, Osborn J. Offset analgesia is mediated by activation in the region of the periaqueductal grey and rostral ventromedial medulla. *Neuroimage 47*:1002–6, 2009; Yelle MD, Oshiro Y, Kraft RA, Coghill RC. Temporal filtering of nociceptive information by dynamic activation of endogenous pain modulatory systems. *J Neuroscience 29*:10264–71, 2009; Ruscheweyh R, Kühnel M, Filippopulos F, Blum B, Eggert T, and Straube A. Altered experimental pain perception after cerebellar infarction. *Pain 155*: 1303–1312, 2014. Porreca F, and Navratilova E. Reward, motivation, and emotion of pain and its relief. *Pain 158* Suppl 1: S43–S49, 2017.

21. Derbyshire SW, Osborn J. Offset analgesia is mediated by activation in the region of the periaqueductal grey and rostral ventromedial medulla. *NeuroImage 47*:1002–6, 2009; Yelle MD, Oshiro Y, Kraft RA, Coghill RC. Temporal filtering of nociceptive information by dynamic activation of endogenous pain modulatory systems. *J Neuroscience 29*:10264–71, 2009; Ruscheweyh R, Kühnel M, Filippopulos F, Blum B, Eggert T, and Straube A. Altered experimental pain perception after cerebellar infarction. *Pain 155*: 1303–1312, 2014; Porreca F, and Navratilova E. Reward, motivation, and emotion of pain and its relief. *Pain 158* Suppl 1: S43–S49, 2017.

22. From the *Merriam-Webster Dictionary*: 1 a: a usually pharmacologically inert preparation prescribed more for the mental relief of the patient than for its actual effect on a disorder; b: an inert or innocuous substance used especially in controlled experiments testing the efficacy of another substance (as a drug). 2: something tending to soothe. See: Wall PD. Pain and the placebo response. *Ciba Foundation Symposium 174*: 187–211, 1993, for a prescient discussion of placebo neurobiology before the surge in functional imaging studies.

23. Haake M, Muller HH, Schade-Brittinger C, Basler HD, Schafer H, Maier C, Endres HG, Trampisch HJ, and Molsberger A. German Acupuncture Trials (GERAC) for chronic low back pain: Randomized, multicenter, blinded, parallel-group trial with 3 groups. *Archives of Internal Medicine 167*: 1892–1898, 2007.

24. Jensen KB, Kaptchuk TJ, Kirsch I, Raicek J, Lindstrom KM, Berna C, Gollub RL, Ingvar M, and Kong J. Nonconscious activation of placebo and nocebo pain responses. *Proceedings of the National Academy of Sciences USA 109*: 15959–15964, 2012; Petersen GL, Finnerup NB, Colloca L, Amanzio M, Price DD, Jensen TS, and Vase L. The magnitude of nocebo effects in pain: A meta-analysis. *Pain 155*: 1426–1434, 2014; See Table 2 in: Sullivan GM, and Feinn R. Using effect size—or why the P value is not enough. *Journal of Graduate Medical Education 4*: 279–282, 2012.

25. Levine JD, Gordon NC, and Fields HL. Naloxone dose dependently produces analgesia and hyperalgesia in postoperative pain. *Nature 278*: 740–741, 1979; Levine JD, Gordon NC, Jones RT, and Fields HL. The narcotic antagonist naloxone enhances clinical pain. *Nature 272*: 826–827, 1978.

26. Gracely RH, Dubner R, Wolskee PJ, and Deeter WR. Placebo and naloxone can alter post-surgical pain by separate mechanisms. *Nature 306*: 264–265, 1983; Levine JD, and Gordon NC. Influence of the method of drug administration on analgesic response. *Nature 312*: 755–756, 1984.

27. Casey KL, Svensson P, Morrow TJ, Raz J, Jone C, and Minoshima S. Selective opiate modulation of nociceptive processing in the human brain. *Journal of Neurophysiology 84*: 525–533, 2000; Zubieta JK, Smith YR, Bueller JA, Xu Y, Kilbourn MR, Jewett DM, Meyer CR, Koeppe RA, and Stohler CS. Regional mu opioid receptor regulation of sensory and affective dimensions of pain. *Science 293*: 311–315, 2001; Petrovic P, Kalso E, Petersson KM, and Ingvar M. Placebo and opioid analgesia: Imaging a shared neuronal network. *Science 295*: 1737–1740, 2002.

28. Friston KJ, Harrison L, and Penny W. Dynamic causal modelling. *NeuroImage 19*: 1273–1302, 2003; Deshpande G, and Hu X. Investigating effective brain connectivity from fMRI data: Past findings and current issues with reference to Granger causality analysis. *Brain Connectivity 2*: 235–245, 2012.

29. Wager TD, Rilling JK, Smith EE, Sokolik A, Casey KL, Davidson RJ, Kosslyn SM, Rose RM, and Cohen JD. Placebo-induced changes in fMRI in the anticipation and experience of pain. *Science 303*: 1162–1167, 2004; Benedetti F, Mayberg HS, Wager TD, Stohler CS, and Zubieta JK. Neurobiological mechanisms of the placebo effect. *Journal of Neuroscience 25*: 10390–10402, 2005; Bingel U, Lorenz J, Schoell E, Weiller C, and Buchel C. Mechanisms of placebo analgesia: rACC recruitment of a subcortical antinociceptive network. *Pain 120*: 8–15, 2006; Price DD, Craggs J, Verne GN, Perlstein WM, and Robinson ME. Placebo analgesia is accompanied by large reductions in pain-related brain activity in irritable bowel syndrome patients. *Pain 127*: 63–72, 2007; Eippert F, Bingel U, Schoell ED, Yacubian J, Klinger R, Lorenz J, and Buchel C. Activation of the opioidergic descending pain control system underlies placebo analgesia. *Neuron 63*: 533–543, 2009; Eippert F, Finsterbusch J, Bingel U, and Buchel C. Direct evidence for spinal cord involvement in placebo analgesia. *Science 326*: 404, 2009; Matre D, Casey KL, and Knardahl S. Placebo-induced changes in spinal cord pain processing. *Journal of Neuroscience 26*: 559–563, 2006; Petrovic P, Kalso E, Petersson KM, Andersson J, Fransson P, and Ingvar M. A prefrontal non-opioid mechanism in placebo analgesia. *Pain 150*: 59–65, 2010; Freeman S, Yu R, Egorova N, Chen X, Kirsch I, Claggett B, Kaptchuk TJ, Gollub RL, and Kong J. Distinct neural representations of placebo and nocebo effects. *NeuroImage 112*: 197–207, 2015.

30. Bushnell MC, Ceko M, and Low LA. Cognitive and emotional control of pain and its disruption in chronic pain. *Nature Reviews Neuroscience 14*: 502–511, 2013; Wiech K, Ploner M, and Tracey I. Neurocognitive aspects of pain perception. *Trends in Cognitive Sciences 12*: 306–313, 2008.; Wiech K, Farias M, Kahane G, Shackel N, Tiede W, and Tracey I. An fMRI study measuring analgesia enhanced by religion as a belief system. *Pain 139*: 467–476, 2008.

31. Zeidan F, Martucci KT, Kraft RA, Gordon NS, McHaffie JG, and Coghill RC. Brain mechanisms supporting the modulation of pain by mindfulness meditation. *Journal of Neuroscience 31*: 5540–5548, 2011; Zeidan F, Emerson NM, Farris SR, Ray JN, Jung Y, McHaffie JG, and Coghill RC. Mindfulness Meditation-Based Pain Relief Employs Different Neural Mechanisms than Placebo and Sham Mindfulness Meditation-Induced Analgesia. *Journal of Neuroscience 35*: 15307–15325, 2015.

32. Colloca L, Klinger R, Flor H, and Bingel U. Placebo analgesia: Psychological and neurobiological mechanisms. *Pain 154*: 511–514, 2013.

33. Institute of Medicine. *Relieving Pain in America: A Blueprint for Transforming Prevention, Care, Education, and Research*. Washington, DC: National Academies Press, 2011; Gaskin DJ, and Richard P. The economic costs of pain in the United States. *Journal of Pain 13*: 715–724, 2012.; Forman J. *A Nation in Pain*. New York: Oxford University Press, 2014, p. 464.

34. Merskey H, and Bogduk N. *Classification of Chronic Pain: Descriptions of Chronic Pain Syndromes and Definitions of Pain Terms*. Seattle: IASP Press, 1994, p. 222.

35. Staud R, Craggs JG, Robinson ME, Perlstein WM, and Price DD. Brain activity related to temporal summation of C-fiber evoked pain. *Pain 129*: 130–142, 2007.

36. Casey KL, Morrow TJ, Lorenz J, and Minoshima S. Temporal and spatial dynamics of human forebrain activity during heat pain: Analysis by positron emission tomography. *Journal of Neurophysiology 85*: 951–959, 2001; Tran TD, Wang H, Tandon A, Hernandez-Garcia

L, and Casey KL. Temporal summation of heat pain in humans: Evidence supporting thalamocortical modulation. *Pain 150*: 93–102, 2010.

37. Porro CA, Cettolo V, Francescato MP, and Baraldi P. Temporal and intensity coding of pain in human cortex. *Journal of Neurophysiology 80*: 3312–3320, 1998; Owen DG, Clarke CF, Ganapathy S, Prato FS, and St. Lawrence KS. Using perfusion MRI to measure the dynamic changes in neural activation associated with tonic muscular pain. *Pain 148*: 375–386, 2010.

38. See also the discussion of *long-term potentiation* in: Willis WD Jr, Zhang X, Honda CN, and Giesler GJ Jr. A critical review of the role of the proposed VMpo nucleus in pain. *Journal of Pain 3*: 79–94, 2002..

39. Gracely RH, Lynch SA, and Bennett GJ. Painful neuropathy: Altered central processing maintained dynamically by peripheral input. *Pain 51*: 175–194, 1992; Haroutounian S, Nikolajsen L, Bendtsen TF, Finnerup NB, Kristensen AD, Hasselstrøm JB, and Jensen TS. Primary afferent input critical for maintaining spontaneous pain in peripheral neuropathy. *Pain 155*: 1272–1279, 2014; Vaso A, Adahan H-M, Gjika A, Zahaj S, Zhurda T, Vyshka G, and Devor M. Peripheral nervous system origin of phantom limb pain. *Pain 155*: 1384–1391, 2014.

40. Katz J, and Melzack R. Pain "memories" in phantom limbs: Review and clinical observations. *Pain 43*: 319–336, 1990; Flor H, Elbert T, Knecht S, Wienbruch C, Pantev C, Birbaumer N, Larbig W, and Taub E. Phantom-limb pain as a perceptual correlate of cortical reorganization following arm amputation. *Nature 375*: 482–484, 1995; Ramachandran VS, and Hirstein W. The perception of phantom limbs: The D. O. Hebb lecture. *Brain 121*: 1603–1630, 1998.

41. Vaso A, Adahan H-M, Gjika A, Zahaj S, Zhurda T, Vyshka G, and Devor M. Peripheral nervous system origin of phantom limb pain. *Pain 155*: 1384–1391, 2014.

42. Nathan PW, Noordenbos W, and Wall PD. Ongoing activity in peripheral nerve: Interactions between electrical stimulation and ongoing activity. *Experimental Neurology 38*: 90–98, 1973.

43. Chan BL, Witt R, Charrow AP, Magee A, Howard R, Pasquina PF, Heilman KM, and Tsao JW. Mirror therapy for phantom limb pain. *New England Journal of Medicine 357*: 2206–2207, 2007; Diers M, Christmann C, Koeppe C, Ruf M, and Flor H. Mirrored, imagined and executed movements differentially activate sensorimotor cortex in amputees with and without phantom limb pain. *Pain 149*: 296–304, 2010.

44. Institute of Medicine. *Relieving Pain in America: A Blueprint for Transforming Prevention, Care, Education, and Research*. Washington, DC: National Academies Press, 2011.

45. Apkarian AV, Hashmi JA, and Baliki MN. Pain and the brain: Specificity and plasticity of the brain in clinical chronic pain. *Pain 152*: S49–S64, 2011.

46. Baliki MN, Geha PY, Apkarian AV, and Chialvo DR. Beyond feeling: Chronic pain hurts the brain, disrupting the default-mode network dynamics. *Journal of Neuroscience 28*: 1398–1403, 2008.

47. Erpelding N, Moayedi M, and Davis KD. Cortical thickness correlates of pain and temperature sensitivity. *Pain 153*: 1602–1609, 2012; Emerson NM, Zeidan F, Lobanov OV, Hadsel MS, Martucci KT, Quevedo AS, Starr CJ, Nahman-Averbuch H, Weissman-Fogel I, Granovsky Y, Yarnitsky D, and Coghill RC. Pain sensitivity is inversely related to regional grey matter density in the brain. *Pain 155*: 566–573, 2014.

48. Teutsch S, Herken W, Bingel U, Schoell E, and May A. Changes in brain gray matter due to repetitive painful stimulation. *NeuroImage 42*: 845–849, 2008.

49. Apkarian AV, Sosa Y, Sonty S, Levy RM, Harden RN, Parrish TB, and Gitelman DR. Chronic back pain is associated with decreased prefrontal and thalamic gray matter density. *Journal of Neuroscience 24*: 10410–10415, 2004; Apkarian AV, Baliki MN, and Geha PY. Towards a theory of chronic pain. *ProgNeurobiol 87*: 81–97, 2009; Apkarian AV, Hashmi JA, and Baliki MN. Pain and the brain: Specificity and plasticity of the brain in clinical chronic pain. *Pain 152*: S49–S64, 2011; for a recent review, see: Seminowicz DA, and Moayedi M. The dorsolateral prefrontal cortex in acute and chronic pain. *Journal of Pain 18*: 1027–1035, 2017.

50. Alshelh Z, Di Pietro F, Youssef AM, Reeves JM, Macey PM, Vickers ER, Peck CC, Murray GM, and Henderson LA. Chronic Neuropathic Pain: It's about the Rhythm. *Journal of Neuroscience 36*: 1008–1018, 2016; Henderson LA, Peck CC, Petersen ET, Rae CD, Youssef AM, Reeves JM, Wilcox SL, Akhter R, Murray GM, and Gustin SM. Chronic pain: Lost inhibition? *Journal of Neuroscience 33*: 7574–7582, 2013; for a comprehensive review of changes in cognitive modulation during chronic pain, see: Bushnell MC, Ceko M, and Low LA. Cognitive and emotional control of pain and its disruption in chronic pain. *Nature Reviews Neuroscience 14*: 502–511, 2013.

51. Smallwood RF, Laird AR, Ramage AE, Parkinson AL, Lewis J, Clauw DJ, Williams DA, Schmidt-Wilcke T, Farrell MJ, Eickhoff SB, and Robin DA. Structural brain anomalies and chronic pain: A quantitative meta-analysis of gray matter volume. *Journal of Pain 14*: 663–675, 2013.

52. Davis KD, Flor H, Greely HT, Iannetti GD, Mackey S, Ploner M, Pustilnik A, Tracey I, Treede R-D, and Wager TD. Brain imaging tests for chronic pain: Medical, legal and ethical issues and recommendations. *Nature Reviews Neurology 13*: 624–638, 2017.

Chapter 11

1. Compton WM, and Volkow ND. Major increases in opioid analgesic abuse in the United States: Concerns and strategies. *Drug and Alcohol Dependence 81*: 103–107, 2006. See also: http://www.cdc.gov/vitalsigns (November 2011).

2. The international classification of headache disorders, 3rd edition (beta version). *Cephalalgia 33*: 629–808, 2013.

3. Akerman S, Holland PR, and Goadsby PJ. Diencephalic and brainstem mechanisms in migraine. *Nature Reviews Neuroscience 12*: 570–584, 2011; Goadsby PJ, Charbit AR, Andreou AP, Akerman S, and Holland PR. Neurobiology of migraine. *Neuroscience 161*: 327–341, 2009; Goadsby PJ, Lipton RB, and Ferrari MD. Migraine: Current understanding and treatment. *New England Journal of Medicine 346*: 257–270, 2002. For a discussion of migraine genetics and the mechanism of migraine aura, see: Moskowitz MA. Deciphering migraine mechanisms: Clues from familial hemiplegic migraine genotypes. *Annals of Neurology 55*: 276–280, 2004; Burstein R, Cutrer MF, and Yarnitsky D. The development of cutaneous allodynia during a migraine attack clinical evidence for the sequential recruitment of spinal and supraspinal nociceptive neurons in migraine. *Brain 123*: 1703–1709, 2000; Burstein R, Yarnitsky D, Goor-Aryeh I, Ransil BJ, and Bajwa ZH. An association between migraine and cutaneous allodynia. *Annals of Neurology 47*: 614–624, 2000.

4. Burstein R, Cutrer MF, and Yarnitsky D. The development of cutaneous allodynia during a migraine attack clinical evidence for the sequential recruitment of spinal and supraspinal nociceptive neurons in migraine. *Brain 123*: 1703–1709, 2000; Burstein R, Yarnitsky D, Goor-Aryeh I, Ransil BJ, and Bajwa ZH. An association between migraine and cutaneous allodynia. *Annals of Neurology 47*: 614–624, 2000.

5. Fumal A, and Schoenen J. Tension-type headache: Current research and clinical management. *Lancet Neurol 7*: 70–83, 2008.
6. Mo J, Maizels M, Ding M, and Ahn AH. Does throbbing pain have a brain signature? *Pain 154*: 1150–1155, 2013; Goadsby PJ. All that is obvious is not clear: What is the origin of throbbing pain in migraine? *Pain 154*: 970–971, 2013; Maniyar FH, and Goadsby PJ. Functional imaging in chronic migraine. *Current Pain and Headache Reports 17*: 333, 2013; Goadsby PJ. The vascular theory of migraine: A great story wrecked by the facts. *Brain 132*: 6–7, 2009; Schytz HW, Birk S, Wienecke T, Kruuse C, Olesen J, and Ashina M. PACAP38 induces migraine-like attacks in patients with migraine without aura. *Brain 132*: 16–25, 2009. See also: Akerman S, Holland PR, and Goadsby PJ. Diencephalic and brainstem mechanisms in migraine. *Nature Reviews Neuroscience 12*: 570–584, 2011..
7. Kroger IL, and May A. Triptan-induced disruption of trigemino-cortical connectivity. *Neurology 84*: 2124–2131, 2015; Goadsby PJ. Comment: How do triptans work in migraine? *Neurology 84*: 2129, 2015.
8. Ramachandran R, and Yaksh TL. Therapeutic use of botulinum toxin in migraine: Mechanisms of action. *British Journal of Pharmacology 171*: 4177–4192, 2014.
9. Akerman S, Holland PR, and Goadsby PJ. Diencephalic and brainstem mechanisms in migraine. *Nature Reviews Neuroscience 12*: 570–584, 2011; Iyengar S, Ossipov MH, and Johnson KW. The role of calcitonin gene-related peptide in peripheral and central pain mechanisms including migraine. *Pain 158*: 543–559, 2017.
10. Langemark M, Jensen K, Jensen TS, and Olesen J. Pressure pain thresholds and thermal nociceptive thresholds in chronic tension-type headache. *Pain 38*: 203–210, 1989; Schmidt-Hansen PT, Svensson P, Bendtsen L, Graven-Nielsen T, and Bach FW. Increased muscle pain sensitivity in patients with tension-type headache. *Pain 129*: 113–121, 2007; Buchgreitz L, Lyngberg AC, Bendtsen L, and Jensen R. Increased pain sensitivity is not a risk factor but a consequence of frequent headache: A population-based follow-up study. *Pain 137*: 623–630, 2008.
11. Milner B, Squire LR, and Kandel ER. Cognitive neuroscience and the study of memory. *Neuron 20*: 445–468, 1998.
12. Craig AD. Pain mechanisms: Labeled lines versus convergence in central processing. *Annual Review of Neuroscience 26*: 1–30, 2003; Craig AD. How do you feel—now? The anterior insula and human awareness. *Nature Reviews Neuroscience 10*: 59–70, 2009; Craig AD. The sentient self. *Brain Structure and Function 214*: 563–577, 2010.
13. Damasio A, Damasio H, and Tranel D. Persistence of feelings and sentience after bilateral damage of the insula. *Cerebral Cortex 23*: 833–846, 2013.
14. Adolphs R, Damasio H, Tranel D, Cooper G, and Damasio AR. A role for somatosensory cortices in the visual recognition of emotion as revealed by three-dimensional lesion mapping. *Journal of Neuroscience 20*: 2683–2690, 2000. See also: Feinstein JS. Lesion studies of human emotion and feeling. *Current Opinion in Neurobiology 23*: 304–309, 2013.
15. LeDoux J. Rethinking the emotional brain. *Neuron 73*: 653–676, 2012; Salamone JD. The involvement of nucleus accumbens dopamine in appetitive and aversive motivation. *Behavioural Brain Research 61*: 117–133, 1994; Berridge KC, and Kringelbach ML. Neuroscience of affect: Brain mechanisms of pleasure and displeasure. *Current Opinion in Neurobiology 23*: 294–303, 2013. For a discussion of pain as a primordial emotion, see: Denton DA. *The Primordial Emotions: The Dawning of Consciousness*. New York: Oxford University Press, 2005, pp. 162–165.
16. Feinstein JS, Rudrauf D, Khalsa SS, Cassell MD, Bruss J, Grabowski TJ, and Tranel D. Bilateral limbic system destruction in man. *Journal of Clinical and Experimental*

Neuropsychology 32: 88–106, 2010; Khalsa SS, Rudrauf D, Feinstein JS, and Tranel D. The pathways of interoceptive awareness. *Nature Neuroscience 12*: 1494–1496, 2009; Philippi CL, Feinstein JS, Khalsa SS, Damasio A, Tranel D, Landini G, Williford K, and Rudrauf D. Preserved self-awareness following extensive bilateral brain damage to the insula, anterior cingulate, and medial prefrontal cortices. *PLoS ONE 7*: e38413, 2012.

17. Starr CJ, Sawaki L, Wittenberg GF, Burdette JH, Oshiro Y, Quevedo AS, and Coghill RC. Roles of the insular cortex in the modulation of pain: Insights from brain lesions. *Journal of Neuroscience 29*: 2684–2694, 2009.

18. Craig AD (Bud). *How Do You Feel? An Interoceptive Moment with Your Neurobiological Self.* Princeton, NJ: Princeton University Press, 2015, p. 343; Gu X, Gao Z, Wang X, Liu X, Knight RT, Hof PR, and Fan J. Anterior insular cortex is necessary for empathetic pain perception. *Brain 135*: 2726–2735, 2012; Gu X, Hof PR, Friston KJ, and Fan J. Anterior insular cortex and emotional awareness. *Journal of Comparative Neurology 521*: 3371–3388, 2013; Ibanez A, Gleichgerrcht E, and Manes F. Clinical effects of insular damage in humans. *Brain Structure and Function 214*: 397–410, 2010.

19. Damasio A, Damasio H, and Tranel D. Persistence of feelings and sentience after bilateral damage of the insula. *Cerebral Cortex 23*: 833–846, 2013; Philippi CL, Feinstein JS, Khalsa SS, Damasio A, Tranel D, Landini G, Williford K, and Rudrauf D. Preserved self-awareness following extensive bilateral brain damage to the insula, anterior cingulate, and medial prefrontal cortices. *PLoS ONE 7*: e38413, 2012; see also: Shackman AJ, Salomons TV, Slagter HA, Fox AS, Winter JJ, and Davidson RJ. The integration of negative affect, pain and cognitive control in the cingulate cortex. *Nature Reviews Neuroscience 12*: 154–167, 2011. This latter study presents evidence that the pain-responsive part of the anterior cingulate cortex integrates nociceptive, affective, and cognitive information to organize defensive behaviors. Most of the bilateral anterior cingulate lesion patients extensively studied by Cohen et al. (Cohen RA, Kaplan RF, Moser DJ, Jenkins MA, and Wilkinson H. Impairments of attention after cingulotomy. *Neurology 53*: 819–824, 1999.) had persistent cognitive deficits (attention, response selection) and affective blunting (less bothered by pain) consistent with that integrative interpretation. Unlike the patient of Damasio et al., however, the responses of the patients described by Cohen et al. had *chronic, not acute,* pain; this could be an important difference in interpreting the effect of cingulate cortex lesions.

20. Papez JW. A proposed mechanism of emotion. *Archives of Neurological Psychiatry 38*: 725–743, 1937; MacLean PD. Psychosomatic disease and the "visceral brain." *Psychosomatic Medicine 11*: 338–353, 1949.

21. Bard P. A diencephalic mechanism for the expression of rage with special reference to the sympathetic nervous system. *American Journal of Physiology 84*: 490–515, 1928.

22. Sebel PS, Bowdle TA, Ghoneim MM, Rampil IJ, Padilla RE, Gan TJ, and Domino KB. The incidence of awareness during anesthesia: A multicenter United States study. *Anesthesia Analgesia 99*: 833–839, 2004.

23. Apfelbaum JL, et al. Practice advisory for intraoperative awareness and brain function monitoring: A report by the American Society of Anesthesiologists Task Force on Intraoperative Awareness. *Anesthesiology 104*: 847–864, 2006.

24. Brice DD, Hetherington RR, and Utting JE. A simple study of awareness and dreaming during anaesthesia. *British Journal of Anaesthesia 42*: 535–542, 1970.

25. For a discussion of the use of EEG and of evoked potentials during anesthesia, see: Schneider G. Monitoring anesthetic depth. In: Mashour GA (Ed.), *Consciousness, Awareness, and Anesthesia.* New York: Cambridge University Press, 2010, pp. 114–130.

26. Avidan MS, Jacobsohn E, Glick D, Burnside BA, Zhang L, Villafranca A, Karl L, Kamal S, Torres B, O'Connor M, Evers AS, Gradwohl S, Lin N, Palanca BJ, Mashour GA, and BAG-RR Group. Prevention of intraoperative awareness in a high-risk surgical population. *New England Journal of Medicine 365*: 591–600, 2011. However, see also: Johansen JW, and Sebel PS. Development and clinical application of electroencephalographic bispectrum monitoring. *Anesthesiology 93*: 1336–1344, 2000.

27. Ishizawa Y. Mechanisms of anesthetic actions and the brain. *Journal of Anesthesia 21*: 187–199, 2007.

28. Buzśaki G, and Wang XJ. Mechanisms of gamma oscillations. *Annual Review of Neuroscience 35*: 203–225, 2012; Gross J, Schnitzler A, Timmermann L, and Ploner M. Gamma oscillations in human primary somatosensory cortex reflect pain perception. *PloS Biology 5*: e133, 2007; Hauck M, Lorenz J, and Engel AK. Attention to painful stimulation enhances gamma-band activity and synchronization in human sensorimotor cortex. *Journal of Neuroscience 27*: 9270–9277, 2007; Salinas E, and Sejnowski TJ. Correlated neuronal activity and the flow of neural information. *Nature Reviews Neuroscience 2*: 539–550, 2001; Tiemann L, May ES, Postorino M, Schulz E, Nickel MM, Bingel U, and Ploner M. Differential neurophysiological correlates of bottom-up and top-down modulations of pain. *Pain 156*: 289–296, 2015; Zhang ZG, Hu L, Hung YS, Mouraux A, and Iannetti GD. Gamma-band oscillations in the primary somatosensory cortex: A direct and obligatory correlate of subjective pain intensity. *Journal of Neuroscience 32*: 7429–7438, 2012.

29. Schneider G. Monitoring anesthetic depth. In: Mashour GA (Ed.), *Consciousness, Awareness, and Anesthesia*. New York: Cambridge University Press, 2010, pp. 114–130.

30. Beaumont JG, and Kenealy PM. Incidence and prevalence of the vegetative and minimally conscious states. *Neuropsychological Rehabilitation 15*: 184–189, 2005. The numbers in the main text are calculated on the assumption of 230 million adults in the United States (2015 Census), using the rate estimates given in this article. The number of children in the VS is less certain.

31. Lepore J. *The Politics of Death*. In: The New Yorker. New York: Advance Magazine Publishers Inc., Conde Nast Publications, 2009, pp. 60–67.

32. Schnakers C, Cammille C, Vanhaudenhuyse A, Majerus S, Ledoux D, Boly M, Bruno MA, Boveroux P, Demertzi A, Moonen G, and Laureys S. The Nociception Coma Scale: A new tool to assess nociception in disorders of consciousness. *Pain 148* 215–219, 2010; Chatelle C, Majerus S, Whyte J, Laureys S, and Schnakers C. A sensitive scale to assess nociceptive pain in patients with disorders of consciousness. *Journal of Neurology, Neurosurgery and Psychiatry 83*: 1233–1237, 2012.

33. Casey KL. Pain and consciousness at the bedside. *Pain 148*: 182–183, 2010.

34. This aspect of consciousness is like the *psychological* aspect as defined by Chalmers (Chalmers DJ. *The Conscious Mind*. New York: Oxford University Press, 1996, p. 414) and as distinct from the *phenomenal* aspect. The former refers to consciousness as identified by or causing observed behavior, while the latter refers to personal experience of self and awareness. Preliminary consciousness, as I use this term, is distinguished from the core consciousness of Damasio by its simplicity and emphasis on observed behavior (Damasio A. *The Feeling of What Happens: Body and Emotion in the Making of Consciousness*. New York: Harcourt Brace, 1999, p. 386.)

In daily life we infer the presence of inner experience (phenomenal) from observing behavior (psychological). By italicizing the passage in the body of text, I emphasize that preliminary consciousness is characterized by complex exploratory interactions with the environment. During preliminary consciousness, CNS activity generates movement and, therefore, sensory input that guides those movements, enabling more complex behaviors and the development (and evolution) of phenomenal (subjective) consciousness. See also: Denton DA. *The Primordial Emotions: The Dawning of Consciousness.* New York: Oxford University Press, 2005, pp. 162–165.

35. Nagel T. What is it like to be a bat? *Philosophical Review 83*: 435–450, 1974.

36. Jennett B, and Plum F. Persistent vegetative state after brain damage. *Lancet 299*: 734–737, 1972; The Multi-Society Task Force on PVS. Medical aspects of the persistent vegetative state. *New England Journal of Medicine 330*: 1499–1508, 1994; Quality Standards Subcommittee of the American Academy of Neurology. Practice parameters: Assessment and management of patients in the persistent vegetative state (summary statement). *Neurology 45*: 1015–1018, 1995; Wijdicks EF, Hijdra A, Young GB, Bassetti CL, Wiebe S, and Quality Standards Subcommittee of the American Academy of Neurology. Practice parameter: Prediction of outcome in comatose survivors after cardiopulmonary resuscitation (an evidence-based review): report of the Quality Standards Subcommittee of the American Academy of Neurology. *Neurology 67*: 203–210, 2006.

37. Horstmann A, Frisch S, Jentzsch RT, Muller K, Villringer A, and Schroeter ML. Resuscitating the heart but losing the brain: Brain atrophy in the aftermath of cardiac arrest. *Neurology 74*: 306–312, 2010; Kinney HC, Korein J, Panigraphy A, Dikkes P, and Goode R. Neuropathological findings in the brain of Karen Ann Quinlan. *New England Journl of Medicine 330*: 1469–1475, 1994; Laureys S. Science and society: death, unconsciousness and the brain. *Nature Reviews Neuroscience 6*: 899–909, 2005.

38. Långsjö JW, Alkire MT, Kaskinoro Kd, Hayama H, Maksimow A, Kaisti KK, Aalto S, Aantaa R, Jääskeläinen SK, Revonsuo A, and Scheinin H. Returning from oblivion: Imaging the neural core of consciousness. *Journal of Neuroscience 32*: 4935–4943, 2012. In this PET study, neuronal activity is identified by the localized increase in blood perfusion in response to the metabolic demands of synaptic activity (see Chapter 9).

39. Boly M, Garrido MI, Gosseries O, Bruno MA, Boveroux P, Schnakers C, Massimini M, Litvak V, Laureys S, and Friston K. Preserved feedforward but impaired top-down processes in the vegetative state. *Science 332*: 858–862, 2011; Crone JS, Schurz M, Höller Y, Bergmann J, Monti M, Schmid E, Trinka E, and Kronbichler M. Impaired consciousness is linked to changes in effective connectivity of the posterior cingulate cortex within the default mode network. *NeuroImage 110*: 101–109, 2015; Qin P, Wu X, Huang Z, Duncan NW, Tang W, Wolff A, Hu J, Gao L, Jin Y, Wu X, Zhang J, Lu L, Wu C, Qu X, Mao Y, Weng X, Zhang J, and Northoff G. How are different neural networks related to consciousness? *Annals of Neurology 78*: 594–605, 2015; Laureys S. Science and society: death, unconsciousness and the brain. *Nature Reviews Neuroscience 6*: 899–909, 2005.

40. Fischer DB, Boes AD, Demertzi A, Evrard HC, Laureys S, Edlow BL, Liu H, Saper CB, Pascual-Leone A, Fox MD, and Geerling JC. A human brain network derived from coma-causing brainstem lesions. *Neurology 87*: 2427–2434, 2016.

41. Bastuji H, Frot M, Perchet C, Magnin M, and Garcia-Larrea L. Pain networks from the inside: Spatiotemporal analysis of brain responses leading from nociception to conscious perception. *Human Brain Mapping* (e-publication 9 July 2016).

42. If the reader wishes to explore further the ancient and persisting question of consciousness and inner experience, there are many excellent avenues of entry to the literature. See: Nagel T. What is it like to be a bat? *Philosophical Review 83*: 435–450, 1974.; (Chalmers DJ. *The Conscious Mind.* New York: Oxford University Press, 1996, pp. 414; Gray J. *Consciousness: Creeping Up on the Hard Problem.* Oxford, UK: Oxford University Press, 2004, p. 341; Macphail EM. *The Evolution of Consciousness.* Oxford, UK: Oxford

University Press, 1998, p. 256; Rose S. *The Future of the Brain: The Promise and Perils of Tomorrow's Neuroscience*. Oxford, UK: Oxford University Press, 2005, p. 344; Searle JR. *Minds, Brains, and Science*. Cambridge, MA: Harvard University Press, 1984, p. 107; Low PA. *The Cambridge Declaration on Consciousness*. In: Panksepp J, Reiss D, Edelman D, Van Swinderen B, Low P, and Koch C (Eds.), *The Francis Crick Memorial Conference on Consciousness in Human and Non-Human Animals*. Cambridge, UK: 2012; Price DD, and Barrell JJ. *Inner Experience and Neuroscience: Merging Both Perspectives*. Cambridge, MA: MIT Press, 2012, p. 345. See also: Mashour GA, and Alkire MT. Evolution of consciousness: Phylogeny, ontogeny, and emergence from general anesthesia. *Proceedings of the National Academy of Sciences USA 110* Suppl 2: 10357–10364, 2013; Denton DA. *The Primordial Emotions: The Dawning of Consciousness*. New York: Oxford University Press, 2005, pp. 162–165.

Chapter 12

1. See Chapter 6 for a discussion of psychophysics and nociceptors. See also: Price DD, Greenspan JD, and Dubner R. Neurons involved in the exteroceptive function of pain. *Pain 106*: 215–219, 2003; Green BG. Temperature perception and nociception. *Journal of Neurobiology 61*: 13–29, 2004.

2. Tracey I. Neuroimaging mechanisms in pain: From discovery to translation. *Pain 158* Suppl 1: S115–S122, 2017.

3. Sommer C, Leinders M, and Uceyler N. Inflammation in the pathophysiology of neuropathic pain. *Pain 159*: 595–602, 2018.

4. Lee J-H, Park C-K, Chen G, Han Q, Xie R-G, Liu T, Ji R-R, and Lee S-Y. A monoclonal antibody that targets a NaV1.7 channel voltage sensor for pain and itch relief. *Cell 157*: 1393–1404, 2014.

5. Raouf R, Quick K, and Wood JN. Pain as a channelopathy. *Journal of Clinical Investigation 120*: 3745–3752, 2010; Waxman SG. Nav1.7, its mutations, and the syndromes that they cause. *Neurology 69*: 505–507, 2007; Denton DA. *The Primordial Emotions: The Dawning of Consciousness*. New York: Oxford University Press, 2005, pp. 162–165; Mashour GA, and Alkire MT. Evolution of consciousness: Phylogeny, ontogeny, and emergence from general anesthesia. *Proceedings of the National Academy of Sciences USA 110* Suppl 2: 10357–10364, 2013.

6. The pain mechanism verbally sketched out here has some resemblance to conceptual models recently proposed by Ron Melzack and by Luis Garcia-Larrea and Roland Peyron. However, the descriptive suggestion I offer here is much more limited and focused on the foregoing evidence for the participation of specific CNS structures discussed in the text. Melzack R. Pain and the neuromatrix in the brain. *Journal of Dental Education 65*: 1378–1382, 2001; Garcia-Larrea L, and Peyron R. Pain matrices and neuropathic pain matrices: A review. *Pain 154*, Suppl 1: S29–S43, 2013.

7. Addiction to opioids is an extensive topic and will not be discussed here. There are opioid drugs that are used both for pain and opioid dependence treatment; in general, these drugs also have abuse potential but somewhat less than those acting exclusively at the classical analgesia mu receptor. The following websites contain information about one of these drugs, buprenorphine, which is used primarily for the management of opioid addiction: www.samhsa.gov/medication-assisted-treatment/treatment/buprenorphine; www.naabt.org/education/pharmacoloy_of_buprenorphine.cfm.

8. Mansour A, Khachaturian H, Lewis ME, Akil H, and Watson SJ. Anatomy of CNS opioid receptors. *Trends in Neurosciences 11*: 308–314, 1988; Baumgartner U, Buchholz HG, Bellosevich A, Magerl W, Siessmeier T, Rolke R, Hohnemann S, Piel M, Rosch F, Wester HJ, Henriksen G, Stoeter P, Bartenstein P, Treede RD, and Schreckenberger M. High opiate receptor binding potential in the human lateral pain system. *NeuroImage 30*: 692–699, 2006; Witta J, Palkovits M, Rosenberger J, and Cox BM. Distribution of nociceptin/orphanin FQ in adult human brain. *Brain Research 997*: 24–29, 2004.

9. For a review of the pharmacology of these drugs, see: Stahl SM, Porreca F, Taylor CP, Cheung R, Thorpe AJ, and Clair A. The diverse therapeutic actions of pregabalin: Is a single mechanism responsible for several pharmacological activities? *Trends in Pharmacological Sciences 34*: 332–339, 2013; Taylor CP. Mechanisms of analgesia by gabapentin and pregabalin: Calcium channel [alpha]2-[delta] [Cav[alpha]2-[delta]] ligands. *Pain 142*: 13–16, 2009.

10. Anderson BJ. Paracetamol (acetaminophen): Mechanisms of action. *Pediatric Anesthesia 18*: 915–921, 2008; Pertwee RG. Targeting the endocannabinoid system with cannabinoid receptor agonists: Pharmacological strategies and therapeutic possibilities. *Philosophical Transactions of the Royal Society of London—Series B: Biological Sciences 367*: 3353–3363, 2012; Pickering G, Esteve V, Loriot MA, Eschalier A, and Dubray C. Acetaminophen reinforces descending inhibitory pain pathways. *Clinical Pharmacology and Therapeutics 84*: 47–51, 2008; Pickering G, Kastler A, Macian N, Pereira B, Valabregue R, Lehericy S, Boyer L, Dubray C, and Jean B. The brain signature of paracetamol in healthy volunteers: A double-blind randomized trial. *Drug Design, Development and Therapy 9*: 3853–3862, 2015; Toussaint K, Yang XC, Zielinski MA, Reigle KL, Sacavage SD, Nagar S, and Raffa RB. What do we (not) know about how paracetamol (acetaminophen) works? *Journal of Clinical Pharmacy and Therapeutics 35*: 617–638, 2010; Makin AJ, Wendon J, Williams R. A 7-year experience of severe acetaminophen-induced hepatotoxicity (1987–1993). *Gastroenterology 109*: 1907–1916, 1995.

11. Law LF, and Sluka KA. How does physical activity modulate pain? *Pain 158*: 369–370, 2017; see also Sommer C, Leinders M, and Uceyler N. Inflammation in the pathophysiology of neuropathic pain. *Pain 159*: 595–602, 2018.

12. Verghese A. *Cutting for Stone*. New York: Alfred A. Knopf, 2009, p. 658. In this highly praised novel, a physician and teacher asks his trainees to identify an emergency treatment that is delivered by ear. The answer is "words of comfort."

13. Kupers R, Faymonville ME, and Laureys S. The cognitive modulation of pain: Hypnosis- and placebo-induced analgesia. *Progress in Brain Research 150*: 251–269, 2005; Lorenz J, and Garcia-Larrea L. Contribution of attentional and cognitive factors to laser-evoked brain potentials *Clinical Neurophysiology 33*: 293–301, 2003; Morley S. Efficacy and effectiveness of cognitive behaviour therapy for chronic pain: Progress and some challenges. *Pain 152*: S99–S106, 2011; Petrovic P, and Ingvar M. Imaging cognitive modulation of pain processing. *Pain 95*: 1–5, 2002; Shackman AJ, Salomons TV, Slagter HA, Fox AS, Winter JJ, and Davidson RJ. The integration of negative affect, pain and cognitive control in the cingulate cortex. *Nature Reviews Neuroscience 12*: 154–167, 2011.

14. Perl ER. Ideas about pain, a historical view. *Nature Reviews Neuroscience 8*: 71–80, 2007; Perl ER. Pain mechanisms: A commentary on concepts and issues. *Progress in Neurobiology 94*: 20–38, 2011. In these historically based reviews of the field, Edward Perl (1926–2014), the codiscoverer of nociceptors, identifies the major issues that continue to drive research on the neurobiology of pain and confronts the difficulty of defining pain in neurobiological terms.

15. Sinclair DC. Cutaneous sensation and the doctrine of specific energy. *Brain 78*: 584–614, 1955; Weddell G. Somesthesis and the chemical senses. *Annual Review of Psychology 6*: 119–136, 1955.
16. It is reasonable to assume that the neurobiology of pain would be the same in humans who have impaired language function but are otherwise healthy. Donald Price and James Barrell argue that inner experiences, including but not limited to pain can be measured, thus providing a quantitative foundation for a science of experiential phenomena. Price DD, and Barrell JJ. *Inner Experience and Neuroscience: Merging Both Perspectives.* Cambridge, MA: MIT Press, 2012, p. 345.
17. Nagel T. What is it like to be a bat? *Philosophical Review 83*: 435–450, 1974.; Striedter GF. *Principles of Brain Evolution.* Sunderland, MA: Sinauer Associates, 2005, p. 436.

APPENDIX

1. For a lucid, highly entertaining, and informative history of the discovery of chemical transmission across synapses, see: Valenstein ES. *The War of the Soups and the Sparks.* New York: Columbia University Press, 2005, p. 256.
2. About 80% of the total energy metabolism of the cerebral cortex according to: Magistretti PJ, Pellerin L, Rothman DL, and Shulman RG. Energy on demand. *Science 283*: 496–497, 1999; Magistretti PJ. Low-cost travel in neurons. *Science 325*: 1349–1351, 2009. See also: Shulman RG, Rothman DL, Behar KL, and Hyder F. Energetic basis of brain activity: Implications for neuroimaging. *Trends in Neurosciences 27*: 489–495, 2004.
3. Complete information about the autonomic nervous system is available in: Jänig W. *The Integrative Action of the Autonomic Nervous System.* Cambridge, UK: Cambridge University Press, 2006, p. 600; Saper CB. The central autonomic nervous system: Conscious visceral perception and autonomic pattern generation. *Annual Review of Neuroscience 25*: 433–469, 2002.
4. Jänig W. *The Integrative Action of the Autonomic Nervous System.* Cambridge, UK: Cambridge University Press, 2006, p. 600.
5. Foreman RD. Mechanisms of cardiac pain. *Annual Review of Physiology 61*: 143–167, 1999.
6. The following references provide an overview of basal ganglia structure and function, including their relationship to pain: Albin RL, Young AB, and Penney JB. The functional anatomy of basal ganglia disorders. *Trends in Neurosciences 12*: 366–375, 1989; Chudler EH, and Dong WK. The role of the basal ganglia in nociception and pain. *Pain 60*: 3–38, 1995; Yelnik J. Functional anatomy of the basal ganglia. *Movement Disorders 17* Suppl 3: S15–S21, 2002; Borsook D, Upadhyay J, Chudler EH, and Becerra L. A key role of the basal ganglia in pain and analgesia: Insights gained through human functional imaging. *Molecular Pain 6*: 27, 2010.
7. Zhang X, Honda CN, and Giesler GJ Jr. Position of spinothalamic tract axons in upper cervical spinal cord of monkeys. *Journal of Neurophysiology 84*: 1180–1185, 2000; Zhang X, Wenk HN, Gokin AP, Honda CN, and Giesler GJ Jr. Physiological studies of spinohypothalamic tract neurons in the lumbar enlargement of monkeys. *Journal of Neurophysiology 82*: 1054–1058, 1999; Zhang X, Wenk HN, Honda CN, and Giesler GJ Jr. Locations of spinothalamic tract axons in cervical and thoracic spinal cord white matter in monkeys. *Journal of Neurophysiology 83*: 2869–2880, 2000; see also (Bernard JF, Bester H, and Besson JM. Involvement of the spino-parabrachio-amygdaloid and -hypothalamic pathways in the autonomic and affective emotional aspects of pain. *Progress in Brain Research 107*: 243–255, 1996.

8. Fishman RA. *Cerebrospinal Fluid in Diseases of the Nervous System.* Philadelphia: W.B. Saunders, 1980, p. 384; Cutler RW, and Spertell RB. Cerebrospinal fluid: A selective review. *Annals of Neurology 11*: 1–10, 1982; Johanson CE, Stopa EG, and McMillan PN. The blood-cerebrospinal fluid barrier: Structure and functional significance. In: Nag S (Ed.), *The Blood-Brain and Other Neural Barriers: Reviews and Protocols.* New York: Humana Press, 2011, pp. 101–131; Benarroch EE. Neurosteroids: Endogenous modulators of neuronal excitability and plasticity. *Neurology 68*: 945–947, 2007; Engelhardt B, and Sorokin L. The blood-brain and the blood-cerebrospinal fluid barriers: function and dysfunction. *Seminars in Immunopathology 31*: 497–511, 2009.

9. Habgood MD, Begley DJ, and Abbott NJ. Determinants of passive drug entry into the central nervous system. *Cellular and Molecular Neurobiology 20*: 231–253, 2000.

10. Tamai I, and Tsuji A. Transporter-mediated permeation of drugs across the blood-brain barrier. *Journal of Pharmaceutical Sciences 89*: 1371–1388, 2000.

11. Bannwarth B, Netter P, Pourel J, Royer RJ, and Gaucher A. Clinical pharmacokinetics of nonsteroidal anti-inflammatory drugs in the cerebrospinal fluid. *Biomedicine and Pharmacotherapy 43*: 121–126, 1989; Bannwarth B, Demotes-Mainard F, Schaeverbeke T, Labat L, and Dehais J. Central analgesic effects of aspirin-like drugs. *Fundamental and Clinical Pharmacology 9*: 1–7, 1995.

12. Beers R, and Camporesi E. Remifentanil update: Clinical science and utility. *CNS Drugs 18*: 1085–1104, 2004;
    Lotsch J, Walter C, Parnham MJ, Oertel BG, and Geisslinger G. Pharmacokinetics of non-intravenous formulations of fentanyl. *Clinical Pharmacokinetics 52*: 23–36, 2013.

13. Stein C, Clark JD, Oh U, Vasko MR, Wilcox GL, Overland AC, Vanderah TW, and Spencer RH. Peripheral mechanisms of pain and analgesia. *Brain Research Reviews 60*: 90–113, 2009.

INDEX

Page references followed by *f*, *t*, or *n* refer to figures, tables, and notes respectively.